The Insulin Resistance Diet
2 week Meal Plan

Louis Laurent

ISBN-10: 1544040555
ISBN-13: 978-1544040554

CONTENTS

INSULIN RESISTANCE DIET

Health experts estimate that in the next 25 years the number of people suffering from diabetes all over the globe will double from around 190 million to about 325 million. It's imperative that we need to pay more attention to our lifestyle choices and habits. It's also important to make some important changes, especially in our diet.

Various researches suggest that excess weight, particularly excess fat around your waist, is the primary cause of insulin resistance. Fortunately, losing excess weight will help the body respond to insulin better.

If you are pre-diabetic or insulin resistant, you can delay or prevent developing diabetes by changing your diet. Together with exercise to lose excess weight

An insulin resistant diet, a diet similar to diabetic meal plan, will not only help you lose weight. Choosing dishes that specifically contain a balanced carbohydrate-protein-and-fat ratio will help regulate the levels of blood glucose and insulin in your body, reducing the risk of developing prediabetes and diabetes.

If you are pre-diabetic or insulin resistant, together with exercise to lose excess weight, following an insulin resistance diet can help delay or prevent developing diabetes.

Changing your diet is not always easy, so here is a meal plan that you can follow for 14 days to start a healthier lifestyle. The recipes in this meal plan are balanced to follow the carbohydrate-protein ratio specifically designed for an insulin resistance diet.

THE 2 WEEK MEAL PLAN

WEEK 1 - DAY 1

Breakfast
Cinnamon Donut Muffins a.k.a Breakfast French Puffs)
Serves: 10
Prep. Time: 10 minutes
Cook Time: 18 minutes

Nutrition Facts per Serving:
Calories 251
Total Fat 16.4g
Total Carbs 18.9g
Protein 9.3g

Lunch
Tunisian-Inspired Tuna Salad
Serves: 6
Prep. Time: 15 minutes

Nutrition Facts per Serving:
Calories 322
Total Fat 18.1g
Total Carbs 28.4g
Protein 13.6g

Snack
Jalapeno Poppers - VEGETARIAN
Serves: 12
Prep. Time: 10 minutes
Cook Time: 20 minutes

Nutrition Facts per Serving:
Calories 242
Total Fat 15.4g

Total Carbs 18.9g
Protein 9.2g

Dinner
Sautéed Vegetables and Salmon
Serves: 4
Prep. Time: 5 minutes
Cook Time: 15 minutes

Nutrition Facts per Serving:
Calories 140
Total Fat 5.0g
Total Carbs 17.0g
Protein 8.5g

WEEK 1 - DAY 2

Breakfast
Breakfast Sticks
Serves: 8
Prep. Time: 20 minutes
Cook Time: 15-20 minutes

Nutrition Facts per Serving:
Calories 267
Total Fat 15.1g
Total Carbs 22.0g
Protein 10.5g

Lunch
5-Minute Egg and Avocado Toast - VEGETARIAN

Serves: 1
Prep. Time: 5 minutes
Cook Time: 5 minutes

Nutrition Facts per Serving:
Calories 392
Total Fat 25.7g
Total Carbs 29.7g
Protein 13.9g

Snack
Chipotle Meatballs
Serves: 12
Prep. Time: 30 minutes
Cook Time: 6-10 minutes

Nutrition Facts per Serving:
Calories 164
Total Fat 9.1g
Total Carbs 14.6g
Protein 7.3g

Dinner
Roasted Cauliflower Salad with Maple-Balsamic Reduction
Serves: 6
Prep. Time: 10 minutes
Cook Time: 25 minutes

Nutrition Facts per Serving:
Calories 201
Total Fat 3.7g
Total Carbs 30.6g
Protein 14.1g

WEEK 1 - DAY 3
Breakfast

Breakfast Calzones
Serves: 4
Prep. Time: 35 minutes
Cook Time: 10-20 minutes

Nutrition Facts per Serving:
Calories 477
Total Fat 32.5g
Total Carbs 32.3g
Protein 13.9g

Lunch
Kale with Stewed Tomatoes, Bacon, and White Beans
Serves: 4-6
Prep. Time: 20 minutes
Cook Time: 10-12 minutes

Nutrition Facts per Serving:
Calories 299
Total Fat 15.4g
Total Carbs 30.3g
Protein 14.2g

Snack
Cheese and Bacon Egg McMuffin-Copy-Cat Cups
Serves: 6
Prep. Time: 25 minutes
Cook Time: 15-20 minutes

Nutrition Facts per Serving:
Calories 275
Total Fat 10.9g
Total Carbs 30.3g
Protein 13.9g

Dinner
Roasted Vegetable Salad and Avocado Dressing
Serves: 4
Prep. Time: 30 minutes
Cook Time: 40 minutes

Nutrition Facts per Serving:
Calories 466
Total Fat 35.9g
Total Carbs 29.7g
Protein 14.0g

WEEK 1 - DAY 4
Breakfast
Breakfast Quesadillas
Serves: 1
Prep. Time: 15 minutes
Cook Time: 5-7 minutes

Nutrition Facts per Serving:
Calories 230
Total Fat 8.5g
Total Carbs 26.6g
Protein 12.8g

Lunch
Green Pea Guacamole Lettuce or Kale Wraps
Serves: 2
Prep. Time: 10 minutes

Nutrition Facts per Serving:
Calories 298
Total Fat 20.4g
Total Carbs 22.1g

Protein 10.5g

Snack
Cheesy Spinach Pinwheels
Serves: 8
Prep. Time: 35 minutes
Cook Time: 20 minutes

Nutrition Facts per Serving:
Calories 139
Total Fat 4.9g
Total Carbs 16.2g
Protein 8.2g

Dinner
Broccoli Mac and Cheese
Serves: 8
Prep. Time: 20 minutes
Cook Time: 10 minutes

Nutrition Facts per Serving:
Calories 311
Total Fat 16.3g
Total Carbs 30.4g
Protein 14.6g

WEEK 1 - DAY 5
Breakfast
Breakfast Casserole
Serves: 12
Prep. Time: 20 minutes
Cook Time: 30 minutes

Nutrition Facts per Serving:
Calories 288

Total Fat 13.1g
Total Carbs 28.3g
Protein 13.6g

Lunch
BLT Filled Avocados
Serves: 8
Prep. Time: 10 minutes

Nutrition Facts per Serving:
Calories 580
Total Fat 50.4g
Total Carbs 25.9g
Protein 12.4g

Snack
Crunchy Crescent Havarti and Ham
Serves: 20
Prep. Time: 10 minutes
Cook Time: 20 minutes

Nutrition Facts per Serving:
Calories 162
Total Fat 6.6g
Total Carbs 17.1g
Protein 8.6g

Dinner
Chicken and Zucchini Fritters with Avocado Dip
Serves: 4
Prep. Time: 20 minutes
Cook Time: 30 minutes

Nutrition Facts per Serving:
Calories 280

Total Fat 13.8g
Total Carbs 29.9g
Protein 14.3g

WEEK 1 - DAY 6

Breakfast
Pomegranate, Feta, and Avocado Toast
Serves: 2
Prep Time: 15 minutes

Nutrition Facts per Serving:
Calories 329
Total Fat 26.9g
Total Carbs 16.5g
Protein 8.3g

Lunch
Basil Tomato Chicken Stew
Serves: 4
Prep. Time: 5 minutes
Cook Time: 20 minutes

Nutrition Facts per Serving:
Calories 204
Total Fat 5.3g
Total Carbs 29.9g
Protein 14.0g

Snack
Jalapeno Meatball Ring
Serves: 8
Prep. Time: 20 minutes
Cook Time: 20 minutes

Nutrition Facts per Serving:
Calories 252
Total Fat 9.8g
Total Carbs 29.9g
Protein 14.2g

Dinner
Chicken Pot Pie
Servings: 8
Prep. Time: 20 min
Cook Time: 20-25 minutes

Nutrition Facts per Serving:
Calories 231
Total Fat 7.4g
Total Carbs 28.0g
Protein 13.5g

WEEK 1 - DAY 7
Breakfast
Spinach, Parmesan, Egg, and Tomato Toast - VEGETARIAN
Serves: 1
Prep. Time: 15 minutes

Nutrition Facts per Serving:
Calories 173
Total Fat 7.1g
Total Carbs 19.1g
Protein 10.5g

Lunch
Cauliflower Broccoli Cheese Sticks -VEGETARIAN
Serves: 4

Prep. Time: 1 hr, 20 minutes
Cook Time: 32 minutes

Nutrition Facts per Serving:
Calories 154
Total Fat 5.2g
Total Carbs 19.8g
Protein 9.8g

Snack
Roasted Asparagus with Shallot Mustard Sauce - VEGETARIAN
Serves: 2
Prep. Time: 10 minutes
Cook Time: 10 minutes

Nutrition Facts per Serving:
Calories 405
Total Fat 33.2g
Total Carbs 23.5g
Protein 11.4g

Dinner
Vegan Lasagna
Serves: 12
Prep. Time: 35 minutes
Cook Time: 60 minutes

Nutrition Facts per Serving:
Calories 271
Total Fat 13.5g
Total Carbs 28.4g
Protein 13.5g

WEEK 2 - DAY 1

Breakfast
Spicy Taquito Breakfast
Serves: 5
Prep. Time: 20 minutes
Cook Time: 15 minutes

Nutrition Facts per Serving:
Calories 329
Total Fat 18.7g
Total Carbs 29.6g
Protein 13.3g

Lunch
Tomato and Avocado Salad
Serves: 2
Prep. Time: 10 minutes

Nutrition Facts per Serving:
Calories 507
Total Fat 40.5g
Total Carbs 29.6g
Protein 14.3g

Snack
Pepperoni Pizza Pretzels
Serves: 6
Prep. Time: 30 minutes
Cook Time: 20 minutes

Nutrition Facts per Serving:
Calories 524
Total Fat 39.3g
Total Carbs 27.8g
Protein 13.1g

Dinner
Tofu Fajitas and Guacamole Crema - VEGETARIAN
Serves: 6
Prep. Time: 10 minutes
Cook Time: 35 minutes

Nutrition Facts per Serving:
Calories 286
Total Fat 19.5g
Total Carbs 22.0g
Protein 10.2g

WEEK 2 - DAY 2
Breakfast
Nutella Pancake Breakfast Pizzas
Serves: 1
Prep. Time: 5 minutes
Cook Time: 5 minutes

Nutrition Facts per Serving:
Calories 384
Total Fat 22.8g
Total Carbs 30.6g
Protein 13.5g

Lunch
Panzanella Lunch
Serves: 2
Prep. Time: 20 minutes

Nutrition Facts per Serving:
Calories 223
Total Fat 8.3g
Total Carbs 25.3g
Protein 12.3g

Snack
Streusel Topped Whole-Wheat Cranberry Apple Muffins
Serves: 12
Prep. Time: 10 minutes
Cook Time: 18-20 minutes

Nutrition Facts per Serving:
Calories 336
Total Fat 21.1g
Total Carbs 24.4g
Protein 12.0g

Dinner
Zucchini Noodles, Shiitake Mushrooms, and Tomato Sauce
Serves: 2
Prep. Time: 10 minutes
Cook Time: 40 minutes

Nutrition Facts per Serving:
Calories 403
Total Fat 28.7g
Total Carbs 29.9g
Protein 14.0g

WEEK 2 - DAY 3
Breakfast
Egg Muffin Breakfast
Serves: 12
Prep. Time: 15 minutes
Cook Time: 20-25 minutes

Nutrition Facts per Serving:
Calories 219

Total Fat 8.5g
Total Carbs 24.3g
Protein 11.6g

Lunch
Zoodle French Onion Bake - VEGETARIAN

Serves: 4
Prep. Time: 15 minutes
Cook Time: 40 minutes

Nutrition Facts per Serving:
Calories 259
Total Fat 15.3g
Total Carbs 20.8g
Protein 10.5g

Snack
Fried Provolone, Crumbled Bacon, and Tomato Sandwich

Serves: 2
Prep. Time: 10 minutes
Cook Time: 20 minutes

Nutrition Facts per Serving:
Calories 297
Total Fat 19.1g
Total Carbs 21.6g
Protein 10.8g

Dinner
Grilled Zucchini and Eggplant Parmesan - VEGETARIAN

Serves: 4
Prep. Time: 20 minutes
Cook Time: 10 minutes

Nutrition Facts per Serving:
Calories 204

Total Fat 11.4g
Total Carbs 20.0g
Protein 10.0g

WEEK 2 - DAY 4
Breakfast
Breakfast Parsnip Hash
Serves: 3
Prep. Time: 20 minutes
Cook Time: 30 minutes

Nutrition Facts per Serving:
Calories 238
Total Fat 9.4g
Total Carbs 27.4g
Protein 12.7g

Lunch
Deviled Egg Finger Sandwiches -VEGETARIAN
Serves: 2
Prep. Time: 10 minutes

Nutrition Facts per Serving:
Calories 304
Total Fat 14.6
Total Carbs 29.9g
Protein 13.7g

Snack
Crusty Herb-Parmesan Zucchini Bites - VEGETARIAN
Serves: 4
Prep. Time: 20 minutes
Cook Time: 15 minutes

Nutrition Facts per Serving:
Calories 111
Total Fat 3.8g
Total Carbs 14.8g
Protein 7.8g

Dinner
Coconut Curry Cauliflower
Serves: 3
Prep. Time: 20 minutes
Cook Time: 20 minutes

Nutrition Facts per Serving:
Calories 580
Total Fat 50.0g
Total Carbs 25.8g
Protein 12.2g

WEEK 2 - DAY 5
Breakfast
Breakfast BLT
Serves: 4
Prep. Time: 10 minutes
Cook Time: 10 minutes

Nutrition Facts per Serving:
Calories 334
Total Fat 20.3g
Total Carbs 26.6g
Protein 12.5g

Lunch
Avocado Chicken Lime Soup
Serves: 6
Prep. Time: 15 minutes

Cook Time: 20 minutes

Nutrition Facts per Serving:
Calories 386
Total Fat 25.3g
Total Carbs 30.1g
Protein 13.9g

Snack
Cauliflower-Gruyere Flatbread
Serves: 4
Prep. Time: 10 min
Cook Time: 5 min

Nutrition Facts per Serving:
Calories 286
Total Fat 12.7
Total Carbs 30.3g
Protein 14.2g

Dinner
Ratatouille
Serves: 4
Prep. Time: 15 minutes
Cook Time: 1 hour

Nutrition Facts per Serving:
Calories 206
Total Fat 8.2g
Total Carbs 24.7g
Protein 11.8g

WEEK 2 - DAY 6
Breakfast
Breakfast Meatballs

Serves: 10
Prep. Time: 20 minutes
Cook Time: 40 minutes

Nutrition Facts per Serving:
Calories 273
Total Fat 14.0g
Total Carbs 25.7g
Protein 12.3g

Lunch
Cheddar Bacon Ranch Pinwheels
Serves: 4
Prep. Time: 10 minutes

Nutrition Facts per Serving:
Calories 447
Total Fat 30.5g
Total Carbs 30.1g
Protein 14.2g

Snack
Honey Drizzled Pistachio and Avocado Bagel Toast
Serves: 1
Prep. Time: 5 minutes

Nutrition Facts per Serving:
Calories 384
Total Fat 24.9g
Total Carbs 28.9g
Protein 13.7g

Dinner
Cauliflower Chicken Fried Rice
Serves: 2
Prep. Time: 25 minutes

Cook Time: 30 minutes

Nutrition Facts per Serving:
Calories 471
Total Fat 35.2g
Total Carbs 30.1g
Protein 14.4g

WEEK 2 - DAY 7
Breakfast
Berry Parfait Breakfast - VEGETARIAN

Serves: 1
Prep. Time: 5 minutes

Nutrition Facts per Serving:
Calories 267
Total Fat 9.8g
Total Carbs 30.2g
Protein 14.0g

Lunch
Avocado Toast and Egg - VEGETARIAN
Serves: 1
Prep. Time: 10 minutes
Cook Time: 10 minutes

Nutrition Facts per Serving:
Calories 383
Total Fat 25.3g
Total Carbs 29.3g
Protein 13.6g

Snack
Cauliflower Hash Browns - VEGETARIAN

Serves: 2
Prep. Time: 30 min
Cook Time: 15 min

Nutrition Facts per Serving:
Calories 279
Total Fat 12.1g
Total Carbs 30.7g
Protein 14.0g

Dinner
Fennel and Roasted Eggplant Pizza - VEGETARIAN
Servings: 4
Prep. Time: 30 minutes
Cook Time: 5 minutes

Nutrition Facts per Serving:
Calories 399
Total Fat 26.2g
Total Carbs 30.7g
Protein 14.4g

BREAKFAST RECIPES

Cinnamon Donut Muffins a.k.a Breakfast French Puffs)

Serves: 10 (1 muffin with 2 1/2 slices cooked bacon per serving)

Prep. Time: 10 minutes

Cook Time: 18 minutes

Nutrition Facts per Serving: Calories 251; Total Fat 16.4g; Saturated Fat 8.0g; Cholesterol 58mg1; Sodium 582mg; Potassium 211mg; Total Carbohydrates 18.9g; Dietary Fiber 2.2g; Sugars 0.7g; Protein 9.3g; Vitamin A 6%; Vitamin C 0%; Calcium 6; Iron 7%

Ingredients:

- 1 1/2 cups flour
- 1 1/2 teaspoon baking powder
- 1 egg
- 1 teaspoon vanilla
- 1/2 cup milk
- 1/2 cup sugar (12 packets stevia)
- 1/2 teaspoon salt
- 1/3 cup butter, softened to room temperature
- 1/4 teaspoon nutmeg
- 2 tablespoons butter, melted, for topping

- Cinnamon and sugar mixture (replace sugar with stevia)
- 2 1/2 slices bacon per serving, cooked, OR 2 1/2 slices ham per serving, cooked

Directions:

1. Put the softened butter in a bowl. Add the sugar and whisk until the mixture is fluffy. Add the egg, milk, and vanilla. Stir in all the dry ingredients until the just moistened
2. Grease 10 muffin cups and fill each 2/3 full with the batter. Bake in a preheated 350F oven for about 18 minutes.
3. After the muffins are baked, while they are still warm, brush each top with melted butter and then roll the muffins in cinnamon-sugar mixture.

Notes: If you are rolling all the muffins in butter, you will need about 1/3 cup. For the cinnamon-sugar mixture, mix about 12 packets stevia and about 1 to 2 teaspoon cinnamon in a shaker.

Breakfast Sticks

Serves: 8 breakfasts sticks (1 stick with 1 pancake)

Prep. Time: 20 minutes

Cook Time: 15-20 minutes

Nutrition Facts per Serving: Calories 267; Total Fat 15.1g; Saturated Fat 4.1g; Cholesterol 138mg; Sodium 477mg; Potassium 164mg; Total Carbohydrates 22.0g;

Protein 10.5g; Vitamin A 6%; Vitamin C 0%; Calcium 21%; and Iron 11%

Ingredients:

- 4 eggs, large-sized, beaten
- 2 slices bacon, chopped
- 2 ounces breakfast sausage
- 2 green onions, large-sized, chopped
- 1 tablespoon oil, your choice
- 1 ounces (1/4 cup) Mozzarella or Monterrey Jack cheese, shredded
- 8 cooked pancakes, homemade or store-bought

Directions:

1. Preheat the oven to 350F. Brush the pan or muffin slots with oil and set aside.
2. In a medium-sized mixing bowl, beat the eggs with the shredded cheese and set aside.
3. In a nonstick skillet, cook the bacon until browned. Add the crumbled sausage in the skillet, cook, stirring frequently, until no longer pink. Add the onion and sauté until the onions start to soften. Remove the skillet from the heat and set aside to cool for about 1-2 minutes.
4. Add the meat mixture into the egg mixture and, using a spoon, beat together.
5. With a measuring 1/4-cup measuring up, scoop 1/4 cup of the batter into each 8 slots.
6. Put into the oven and bake for about 15 to 20 minutes or until the tops are just starting to brown.
7. Meanwhile, cook prepacked pancake mix in a nonstick skillet.
8. With the tip of a knife, remove from the slot or pans. Serve immediately.

Breakfast Calzones
Serves: 4

Prep. Time: 35 minutes

Cook Time: 10-20 minutes

Nutrition Facts per Serving: Calories 477; Total Fat 32.5g; Saturated Fat 9.5g; Cholesterol 178mg; Sodium 613mg; Potassium 146mg; Total Carbohydrates 32.3g; Dietary Fiber 2.6g; Protein 13.9g; Vitamin A 6%; Calcium 8%; and Iron 16%

Ingredients:

- 1/4 cup cheese, shredded
- 300 grams refrigerated pizza dough, homemade or store-bought
- 4 eggs
- 4 slices bacon
- Salt and pepper

Directions:

1. Preheat the oven following the pizza dough instructions.
2. Meanwhile, put 2 sheets paper towel on a microwavable plate. Lay the bacon slices on the paper towels – do not overlap the slices.

Put 2 more paper towels on top of the bacon slices. Heat in for 4-6 minutes in the microwave on HIGH setting. Alternatively, you can cook the bacon in a skillet. If using a skillet, crack the eggs into a bowl and generously season with salt and pepper. Beat and then scramble in the same skillet where the bacon is cooked – remove excess bacon grease from the skillet, leaving only enough oil to cook the eggs.

3. Unroll the pizza dough and, with a rolling pin, roll into 10x12-inch rectangle. Cut the dough vertically into halves and then cut the vertical halves horizontally, making 4 rectangles that are about 5x6-inches.

4. Cut the slices of bacon into halves and put 2 halves into the half portion each rectangle dough. Divide the scrambled eggs into 4 portions and top each portion over the bacon halves. Sprinkle the tops of each with 2 tablespoons cheese. Fold the un-topped portion of each rectangle dough over the cheese and, with a fork, seal each calzone

5. Bake according to the instructions of the pizza dough, or until the calzones are golden. Serve!

Breakfast Quesadillas

Serves: 1

Prep. Time: 15 minutes

Cook Time: 5-7 minutes

Nutrition Facts per Serving: Calories 230; Total Fat 8.5g; Saturated Fat 3.3g; Cholesterol 176mg; Sodium 238mg;Potassium 302mg; Total Carbohydrates 26.6g; Dietary Fiber 3.9g; Sugars 3.6g; Protein 12.8g; Vitamin A 7%; Vitamin C 4%; Calcium 15%; and Iron 9%

Ingredients:

- 5 grams bacon, cooked crispy
- 2 small-sized flour tortillas
- 1 tablespoon sharp cheddar cheese
- 1 egg
- 1 tablespoon yogurt, for serving
- 1 tablespoon salsa, for serving
- Cilantro, for garnish

Directions:

1. In a nonstick skillet, sauté the onions until starting to caramelize. Remove the onions from the skillet and set aside.
2. Whisk the eggs until beaten and cook in the same skillet like an omelet- keeping it flat like a pancake to fit will in the tortilla.
3. Put 1 tortilla on a round Belgian waffle maker. Put the fried eggs, caramelized onions, cheese and bacon on the tortilla. Top with the other tortilla.
4. Close the waffle maker and cook for about 5-7 minutes or until the cheese is completely melted.
5. Remove from the waffle maker and cut into quarters. Garnish with cilantro. Serve with yogurt and salsa. Enjoy!

Breakfast Casserole

Serves: 12 (1 slice of breakfast casserole with 4 slices toasted bread)

Prep. Time: 20 minutes

Cook Time: 30 minutes

Nutrition Facts per Serving: Calories 288; Total Fat 13.1g; Saturated Fat 4.9g; Cholesterol 108mg; Sodium 577mg; Potassium 157mg; Total Carbohydrates 28.3g; Dietary Fiber 1.2g; Sugars 2.8g; Protein 13.6g; Vitamin A 4%; Calcium 17%; and Iron 15%

Ingredients:

- 1 cup cheddar cheese, shredded
- 1 package (8 ounces) crescent rolls
- 1/2 pound mild sausage, crumbled
- 6 eggs, beaten
- 4 slices toasted bread per serving, buttered if desired, for serving

Directions:

1. Preheat the oven to 350F.
2. Grease a 13x9-inch baking dish with nonstick cooking oil.
3. Cook the sausage in a skillet until browned. Transfer into a plate and set aside.
4. Spread the crescent dough into the bottom the baking dish. Add the sausages, spreading evenly over the dough. Pour the beaten eggs over the sausage. Top with the shredded cheese.
5. Bake in the preheated oven for about 30 minutes.
6. When baked, slice into 12 equal-sized pieces. Serve with toasts.

Pomegranate, Feta, and Avocado Toast
Serves: 2 (1 toast with 1 1/2 slices bacon)

Prep. Time: 15 minutes

Nutrition Facts per Serving: Calories 329; Total Fat 26.9g; Saturated Fat 7.7g; Cholesterol 23mg; Sodium 446mg; Potassium 606mg; Total Carbohydrates 16.5g; Dietary Fiber 7.1g; Sugars 3.6g; Protein 8.3g; Vitamin A 4%; Vitamin C 24%; Calcium 10%; and Iron 7%

Ingredients:

- 1 avocado
- 1 ounce feta cheese, crumbled
- 1 tablespoon lemon juice
- 2 slices of your favorite bread, toasted
- 2 tablespoons pomegranate arils
- 3 slices bacon, cooked
- Salt and pepper

Directions:

1. Mash the avocado meat to desired consistency – you can leave a few chunky pieces, if desired. Spread the avocado on both slices of bread.
2. Sprinkle 1/2 ounce feta cheese and 1 tablespoon pomegranate arils over each and then season with salt and pepper.
3. Drizzle each with lemon juice. Serve with bacon.

Spinach, Parmesan, Egg, and Tomato Toast

Serves: 1

Prep. Time: 15 minutes

Nutrition Facts per Serving: Calories 173; Total Fat 7.1g; Saturated Fat 2.5g; Cholesterol 169mg; Sodium 240mg; Potassium 577mg; Total Carbohydrates 19.1g; Dietary Fiber 2.8g; Sugars 6.2g; Protein 10.5g; Vitamin A 34%; Vitamin C 107%; Calcium 10%; and Iron 33%

Ingredients:

- 1 egg, hard-boiled (or cooked to your preference)
- 1 Roma tomato
- 2 slices of your favorite bread, toasted
- 2 teaspoons cheese, grated
- Handful fresh baby spinach
- Olive oil
- Red Pepper Flakes
- Salt and pepper

Directions:

1. Arrange the spinach on both sides of the toasted bread and season with salt and pepper.
2. Top each with a couple slices of tomatoes, cheese, eggs, and season with salt, pepper, red pepper, and drizzle the top of each with olive oil.

Spicy Taquito Breakfast
Serves: 5 (2 rolls each serving)

Prep. Time: 20 minutes

Cook Time: 15 minutes

Nutrition Facts per Serving: Calories 329; Total Fat 18.7g; Saturated Fat 6.0g;

Cholesterol 151mg; Sodium 288mg; Potassium 421mg; Total Carbohydrates 29.6g; Dietary Fiber 5.6g; Sugars 3.8g; Protein 13.3g; Vitamin A 34%; Vitamin C 110%; Calcium 18%; and Iron 12%

Ingredients:

- 1 green bell pepper, diced
- 1/2 cup cheddar cheese, shredded
- 1/2 cup fresh cilantro or parsley
- 1/2 cup milk
- 10 tortillas
- 19 grams bacon, cooked, crumbled
- 2 tablespoons chipotle peppers, minced, with adobo sauce
- 3/4 avocado, cubed
- 4 eggs, large-sized

For the dipping sauce

- 2 tablespoons chipotle spread
- 2 tablespoons mayonnaise

Directions:

1. Preheat the oven to 425F.
2. Heat a large-sized skillet on medium heat. Add the bacon until fat is rendered and crispy. Transfer to a plate and set aside to cool. When cool enough to handle, crumble.
3. Remove excess bacon fat from the skillet, leaving only about 1 tablespoon.
4. In a large-sized bowl, whisk the eggs with the milk, chipotle peppers, and bell pepper. Add the cheddar cheese, whisk again, and season with a small pinch of pepper and salt.
5. Reheat the skillet on medium heat. Pour in the egg mixture and slowly scramble until cooked.
6. Put about 3 tablespoons of scrambled egg into each tortilla, sprinkle with the crumbled bacon, and then roll each tortilla.
7. Line a baking sheet with foil. With the seam side faced down, put the rolled tortilla into the baking sheet. Repeat the process with the remaining tortillas, egg, and crumbled bacon. Lightly grease the top of each rolled tortilla rolls with nonstick cooking spray.

8. Bake in the oven for 15 minutes or until crispy and golden brown.
9. Meanwhile, mix the dipping sauce ingredients until well combines.
10. Serve the taquitos with the dipping sauce, cilantro, and diced avocado.

Nutella Pancake Breakfast Pizzas
Serves: 1

Prep. Time: 5 minutes

Cook Time: 5 minutes

Nutrition Facts per Serving: Calories 384;
Total Fat 22.8g; Saturated Fat 12.4g;

Cholesterol 50mg; Sodium 764mg; Potassium
345mg; Total Carbohydrates 30.6g; Dietary
Fiber 2.0g; Sugars 16.5g; Protein 13.5g;
Vitamin A 2%; Vitamin C 24%; Calcium 12%;
and Iron 13%

Ingredients:

- 1 pancake OR waffle
- 2 fresh strawberries, quartered
- 2 tablespoons Nutella
- 4 slices bacon, cooked

Directions:

1. Toast the pancake/waffle according to the directions on the package.
2. Spread the Nutella on the wide side of the pancake/waffle.
3. Top with the strawberry quarters. Enjoy with cooked bacon.

Egg Muffin Breakfast
Serves: 12 (1 muffin with 1/2 crescent roll)

Prep. Time: 15 minutes

Cook Time: 20-25 minutes

Nutrition Facts per Serving: Calories 219; Total Fat 8.5g; Saturated Fat 2.7g;

Cholesterol 169mg; Sodium 326mg; Potassium 170mg; Total Carbohydrates 24.3g; Dietary Fiber 1.1g; Sugars 3.8g; Protein 11.6g; Vitamin A 21%; Vitamin C 65%; Calcium 12%; and Iron 14%

Ingredients:

- 1 ounce goat cheese
- 1 red bell pepper
- 1 yellow bell pepper
- 1/2 cup spinach
- 12 eggs
- 2 bacon slices, cooked and crumbled
- Cooking spray
- Pinch black pepper
- Pinch sea salt
- 6 crescent rolls, for serving

Equipment:

- 12-cup muffin tin

Directions:

1. Preheat the oven to 350F.
2. Generously grease the muffin cups with cooking spray and set aside.
3. Chop the spinach and bell peppers into 1/4-inch bite-sized pieces.
4. Evenly divide the vegetables between the muffin cups.
5. In a large-sized bowl, whisk the eggs until well beaten and season with pepper and salt to taste.
6. Evenly divide and pour the beaten egg into each muffin cup, filling each about 3/4 full.
7. Divide the cooked bacon and cheese over the top of each muffin.
8. Bake in the oven for about 20 to 25 minutes – the muffins will puff up, but will deflate as soon as they cool down to room temperature.
9. Store for 5 days in the refrigerator.

Breakfast Parsnip Hash
Serves: 3 (1/3 hash with 2 slices toasted bread)

Prep. Time: 20 minutes

Cook Time: 30 minutes

Nutrition Facts per Serving: Calories 238; Total Fat 9.4g; Saturated Fat 2.9g; Cholesterol 123mg; Sodium 476mg; Potassium 654mg; Total Carbohydrates 27.4g; Dietary Fiber 5.7g; Sugars 6.3g; Protein 12.7g; Vitamin A 22%; Vitamin C 32%;

Calcium 10%; and Iron 21%

Ingredients:
- 1 fresh rosemary sprig, chopped (about 1 tablespoon)
- 1/2 yellow onion, diced
- 2 cups mushrooms, sliced
- 2 eggs
- 2 large handfuls greens (kale or spinach)
- 2 parsnips, medium-sized, grated
- 6 slices bacon, diced
- 6 slices bread, toasted
- Salt and pepper, to taste
-

Directions:

1. Chop the bacon, mushrooms, yellow onion, and rosemary, and grate the parsnip.
2. Heat a large-sized pan or a cast-iron skillet on medium heat. Put the bacon in the pan/skillet and cook for about 5 minutes.
3. Add the onion and cook for 8 minutes, occasionally stirring, or until the bacon is just beginning to crisp a bit and the onion is soft.
4. Add the grated parsnips spread across the pan evenly into a thin layer. Cook for about 2 minutes then stir everything to cook all the parsnips. Cook for 3 minutes more.
5. Add the mushrooms, greens, rosemary, and season with pepper and salt. Stir to combine and cook for 5 minutes, occasionally stirring.
6. Create 2 wells in the hash. Crack an egg into each well and cover the pan. Cook covered for about 5 minutes or until the egg whites turn white and set. Serve.

Breakfast BLT
Serves: 4

Prep. Time: 10 minutes

Cook Time: 10 minutes

Nutrition Facts per Serving: Calories 334; Total Fat 20.3g; Saturated Fat 4.7g;

Cholesterol 185mg; Sodium 687mg; Potassium 246mg; Total Carbohydrates 26.6g; Dietary Fiber 2.2g; Sugars 9.8g; Protein 12.5g; Vitamin A 9%; Vitamin C 21%; Calcium 6%; and Iron 16%

Ingredients:

- 8 slices rustic bread, good-quality, buttered and then toasted
- 8 slices bacon
- 4 green lettuce leaves, large-sized
- 4 eggs
- 1/2 cup mayonnaise
- 1 tomato, large-sized, sliced
- 1 tablespoon prepared basil pesto
- 1 3/4 cup blueberries, divided into 4 servings

Directions:

1. Combine the basil pesto and mayonnaise and set aside.
2. In a large-sized skillet, cook the bacon until crispy and browned. Transfer into a plate.
3. Remove excess bacon fat from the skillet, leaving about 2 tablespoons.
4. Carefully crack and open the eggs into the skillet. Cover and cook on very low heat or until the egg whites are set but the yolks are not cooked completely.
5. Spread the basil-mayo spread on each toasted slice of bread.
6. Divide the lettuce, tomato, and bacon between 4 slices of bread and then top each with an egg. Top each with another bread slice. Serve immediately.

Berry Parfait Breakfast
Serves: 1

Prep. Time: 5 minutes

Nutrition Facts per Serving: Calories 267;
Total Fat 9.8g; Saturated Fat 2.3g;

Cholesterol 10mg; Sodium 120mg; Potassium
637mg; Total Carbohydrates 30.2g; Dietary
Fiber 6.1g; Sugars 22.1g; Protein 14.0g;
Vitamin A 4%; Vitamin C 38%; Calcium 36%;
and Iron 11%

Ingredients:

- 1 container (6-ounce) yogurt, French-vanilla
- 1/2 cup fresh blueberries
- 1/3 fresh blackberries
- 12 almonds, toasted

Directions:

1. In a small-sized cup, put in the fresh blueberries.
2. Add 1/2 of the yogurt and then the fresh blackberries.
3. Top with the remaining yogurt.
4. Serve and enjoy with roasted almonds.

Breakfast Meatballs

Serves: 10 (3 meatballs with 3 slices toasted bread)

Prep. Time: 20 minutes

Cook Time: 40 minutes

Nutrition Facts per Serving: Calories 273; Total Fat 14.0g; Saturated Fat 4.4g;

Cholesterol 38mg; Sodium 528mg; Potassium 533mg; Total Carbohydrates 25.7g; Dietary Fiber 3.0g; Sugars 3.6g; Protein 12.3g; Vitamin A 196%; Vitamin C 34%;

Calcium 10%; and Iron 15%

Ingredients:

- 2 pounds ground breakfast sausage
- 1/2 onion
- 1/2 butternut squash
- 1 teaspoon smoked paprika
- 1 teaspoon cinnamon
- 1 sprig rosemary, diced finely
- 1 cup mushrooms (about 4 ounces)
- 3 slices bread per serving, toasted

Directions:

1. Preheat the oven to 375F. Line a large-sized baking sheet or 2 medium-sized baking sheets with parchment paper.
2. Cut the butternut squash into large-sized cubes. Put the cubes into a food processor and chop into small bits. Transfer into a large-sized bowl.
3. Put the mushrooms and onion into the food processor and chop into small bits. Add into the bowl with squash.
4. Add the sausage, cinnamon, paprika, and rosemary into the bowl.
5. With clean hands, combine the ingredients until well mixed.
6. Form the mixture into 30 pieces golf-sized balls. Put the balls into the prepared baking sheet.
7. Bake for about 40 minutes. when baked, let cool for a couple of minutes. Serve with toasted bread.

Biscuit Bun Breakfast
Serves: 8

Prep. Time: 20 minutes

Cook Time: 35 minutes

Nutrition Facts per Serving: Calories 353; Total Fat 19.8g; Saturated Fat 4.8;

Cholesterol 180mg; Sodium 997mg; Potassium 279mg; Total Carbohydrates 29.2g;

Dietary Fiber 0.9g; Sugars 2.6g; Protein 14.4g; Vitamin A 4%; Vitamin C 1%; Calcium 5%; and Iron 16%

Ingredients:

- 1 can (16.3 ounces) refrigerated buttermilk biscuits (I used Pillsbury™ Grands!™ Homestyle)
- 1/2 cup onion, finely chopped
- 1/4 pound pepper bacon
- 8 eggs
- Salt and pepper, to taste

Equipment:

- Jumbo muffin cups or 8 pieces 6-ounce custard cups

Directions:

1. Preheat the oven to 350F.
2. In a 10-inch skillet, cook the bacon on medium-high heat for about 10-12 minutes or until crisp. Transfer into paper towels and crumble.
3. Remove excess grease from the skillet, leaving about 1 tablespoon.
4. Put the onion in the skillet and sauté or about 2 minutes or until softened.
5. In a small-sized bowl, transfer the crumbled bacon and add the softened onion. Mix until combined and set aside.
6. Grease the muffin cups or custard cups with nonstick cooking spray. Divide the dough into 8 equal-sized portions. Put 1 biscuit dough portion into each muffin/custard cup. Press on the center of each dough to, pressing dough 3/4 of the way up against the sides of the muffin/custard cups.
7. Divide the bacon between each cup, putting each portion on the dough well.
8. Crack 1 each into each, making sure to keep the yolks intact and then season the eggs with salt and pepper to taste.
9. Bake in the oven for about 30-25 minutes or until the yolks and egg whites are firm.

To loosen the biscuit buns, run a small-sized knife around each. Serve immediately

LUNCH RECIPES

Cheddar Bacon Ranch Pinwheels
Serves: 4

Prep. Time: 10 minutes

Nutrition Facts per Serving: Calories 447; Total Fat 30.5g; Saturated Fat 17.2g;

Cholesterol 89mg; Sodium 761mg; Potassium 567mg; Total Carbohydrates 30.1g; Dietary Fiber 2.6g; Sugars 15.3g; Protein 14.2g; Vitamin A 27%; Vitamin C 176%;

Calcium 18%; and Iron 17%

Ingredients:

- 8 ounces cream cheese, softened
- 6 pieces bacon, cooked and then chopped
- 3 large-sized or 6 small-sized tortillas
- 12 tablespoons marinara sauce
- 1/4 cup ranch dressing
- 1/2 cup cheddar cheese, finely shredded
- 1 tablespoons chives, minced
- 1/4 cup orange juice, per serving

Directions:

1. In a small-sized mixing bowl, combine the ranch dressing and cream cheese until smooth. Stir in the bacon, cheddar cheese, and chives.
2. Divide the ranch dressing mixture between each tortilla and spread each portion over each.
3. Tightly roll each tortilla and then slice each into 1-inch pinwheels.

Cauliflower and Broccoli Cheese Sticks
Serves: 4

Prep. Time: 1 hour, 20 minutes

Cook Time: 32 minutes

Nutrition Facts per Serving: Calories 154; Total Fat 5.2g; Saturated Fat 1.9g;

Cholesterol 49mg; Sodium 479mg; Potassium 761mg; Total Carbohydrates 19.8g; Dietary Fiber 6.2g; Sugars 8.6g; Protein 9.8g; Vitamin A 14%; Vitamin C 200%; Calcium 8%; and Iron 9%

Ingredients:

- 1 1/2 cups mozzarella cheese, shredded, divided
- 1 1/2 teaspoons Italian seasoning
- 1 cauliflower head OR 5 cups cauliflower, chopped
- 1 egg, large-sized
- 1 tablespoon flour
- 1/4 teaspoon salt
- 3 cups broccoli florets, chopped
- 3/4 cup marinara sauce

Directions:

1. Bring a pot of water to boil. When boiling, add the broccoli and cauliflower. Boil for 5 minutes. Remove the veggies from the pot and drain in a colander. Transfer into a baking sheet lined with paper towel and let rest for about 1 hour to drain off most of the water from the vegetables, replacing the paper towels, if needed.
2. Preheat the oven to 400F. Put the cauliflower and broccoli in a blender. Add the egg, flour, 1 cup cheese, salt, and Italian seasoning. Pulse until the ingredients are well blended.
3. Line a shallow baking pan with parchment paper. Pour the veggie mixture into the prepared baking pan.
4. Bake in the oven for 20 minutes. Remove the pan from the oven and sprinkle the top with the remaining 1/2 cup cheese. Bake for 10 minutes more and then broil for 2 minutes.
5. Let cool for a bit and slice into equal-sized sticks. Serve with marinara sauce.

Avocado Toast and Egg
Serves: 1

Prep. Time: 10 minutes

Cook Time: 10 minutes

Nutrition Facts per Serving: Calories 383; Total Fat 25.3g; Saturated Fat 5.9g;

Trans Fat 0.2g; Cholesterol 165mg; Sodium 258mg; Potassium 770mg; Total Carbohydrates 29.3g; Dietary Fiber 9.2g; Sugars 7.9g; Protein 13.6g; Vitamin A 8%; Vitamin C 111%; Calcium 8%; and Iron 16%

Ingredients:

- 1 egg
- 1 piece bread, whole wheat or sprouted
- 1 tablespoon cottage cheese (I used Hiland Dairy)
- 1/2 avocado, ripe and soft
- Lime wedge
- 1/4 cup fresh squeezed orange juice, for serving

Directions:

1. Toast the bread.
2. In a small bowl, put the cottage cheese and avocado. Smash the avocado and stir to combine. Spread the avocado mixture on the toasted bread.
3. Coat a pan with oil and heat. Gently crack an egg into the pan, reduce the heat to medium, and cook for 2 minutes.
4. Cover the pan with lid and cook the egg for 1 minute more – do not flip the egg.
5. Using a spatula, loosen the sides of the egg and then slide out from the pan into the toast.
6. Season with sea salt and black pepper and, if desired, squeeze with lime juice. Enjoy with orange juice.

Tunisian-Inspired Tuna Salad
Serves: 6

Prep. Time: 15 minutes

Nutrition Facts per Serving: Calories 322; Total Fat 18.1g; Saturated Fat 2.8g;

Trans Fat 0.5g; Cholesterol 6mg; Sodium 347mg; Potassium 414mg; Total Carbohydrates 28.4g; Dietary Fiber 5.1g; Sugars 5.8g; Protein 13.6g; Vitamin A 25%; Vitamin C 80%; Calcium 9%; and Iron 13%

Ingredients:

- 12 slices whole-wheat bread
- 1 tablespoon capers, chopped
- 1 teaspoon ground cumin
- 1 yellow bell pepper, seeded and diced
- 1/2 English cucumber, seeded and diced
- 120 grams canned flaked tuna, drained
- 2 cloves garlic, chopped
- 2 green onions, thinly sliced
- 2 tablespoons black olives, thinly sliced
- 2 tablespoons flat-leaf parsley, chopped
- 2 tablespoons fresh cilantro, chopped
- 2 teaspoons fresh mint, chopped
- 2 tomatoes, seeded and diced
- 6 tablespoons olive oil

- Salt and pepper

Directions:

1. In a bowl, combine all of the ingredients until mixed and season with pepper and salt.
2. Serve immediately sandwiched between 2 slices of bread.

5-Minute Egg and Avocado Toast
Serves: 1

Prep. Time: 5 minutes

Cook Time: 5 minutes

Nutrition Facts per Serving: Calories 392; Total Fat 25.7g; Saturated Fat 5.9g; Trans Fat 0.4g; Cholesterol 164mg; Sodium 304mg; Potassium 672mg; Total Carbohydrates 29.7g; Dietary Fiber 10.2g; Sugars 3.6g; Protein 13.9g; Vitamin A 7%; Vitamin C 17%; Calcium 9%; and Iron 15%

Ingredients:

- 1 egg (hard-boiled for 5 minutes)
- 1 slice (50 grams) wholegrain bread (toast if preferred)
- 1/2 avocado
- Pinch red chili flakes
- Salt and pepper

Directions:

1. Put the egg in a pot of cold water and bring to a boil. When boiling, reduce heat and leave the egg to sit in the pot for 5 minutes.
2. While the egg is boiling, toast the bread to desired doneness.
3. Put the avocado meat into a bowl and coarsely mash, leaving a few chunks.
4. Spread the mashed avocado on the bread or toast. Sprinkle with black pepper and chili flakes. Enjoy.

Kale with Stewed Tomatoes, Bacon, and White Beans
Serves: 4-6

Prep. Time: 20 minutes

Cook Time: 10-12 minutes

Nutrition Facts per Serving: Calories 299; Total Fat 15.4g; Saturated Fat 3.7g; Cholesterol 21mg; Sodium 495mg; Potassium 1384mg; Total Carbohydrates 30.3g; Dietary Fiber 8.3g; Sugars 8.3g; Protein 14.2g; Vitamin A 359%; Vitamin C 283%; Calcium 21%; and Iron 21%

Ingredients:

- 1 can (15 ounces) Cannellini or Northern Beans, drained not rinsed (I used Bush's Reduced Sodium)
- 1 onion, chopped
- 2 cans (15 ounces each) stewed tomatoes
- 2 tablespoons olive oil
- 2 tablespoons red wine vinegar
- 3-4 cloves garlic, chopped
- 6 cups kale, chopped
- 75 grams bacon, cooked and then crumbled, divided into 4 portions
- Salt and pepper

Directions:

1. Put oil in a large-sized pot or braiser and heat on medium heat. Add the garlic and onion in the pot. Sauté for about 1-2 minutes, stirring to prevent the garlic from burning.
2. A little at a time, add the kale into the pot, tossing using tongs, cooking down each batch a little before adding the next so that it fits. Season with pepper and salt and add in the red wine vinegar.
3. Add the beans and stewed tomatoes into the pot and toss gently to combine.
4. Cook for about 10 to 12 minutes or until the kale is completely cooked. Taste seasoning and adjust as desired. Serve!

Basil Tomato Chicken Stew
Serves: 4

Prep. Time: 5 minutes

Cook Time: 20 minutes

Nutrition Facts per Serving: Calories 204; Total Fat 5.3g; Saturated Fat 0.9g; Cholesterol 20mg; Sodium 659mg; Potassium 1421mg; Total Carbohydrates 29.9g; Dietary Fiber 10.0g; Sugars 14.7g; Protein 14.0g; Vitamin A 199%; Vitamin C 130%; Calcium 12%; and Iron 16%

Ingredients:

- 1 can (14 ounces) cannellini beans
- 1 tablespoons olive oil
- 1 teaspoon salt
- 1 white onion, small-sized, chopped
- 1/2 teaspoon black pepper
- 1/4 cup fresh basil, roughly chopped
- 1/4 teaspoon crushed red pepper flakes
- 2 cans (28 ounces each) whole tomatoes (with juices)
- 2 carrots, peeled and diced
- 2 handfuls baby spinach
- 2 stalks celery, diced
- 3/4 cup cooked chicken, shredded

- 4 cloves garlic

Directions:

1. Put the oil in a large-sized stockpot and heat on medium-high heat. Add the celery, carrots, and onion. Sauté for about 7 minutes, occasionally stirring, until the onion is translucent and soft. Add the garlic; sauté for about 1-2 minutes or until fragrant.
2. Add the rest of the ingredients and stir to combine. With a long spoon, crush the tomatoes. Bring the mixture to a boil. When boiling, reduce the heat to medium-low and partially cover the pot. Simmer for 10 minutes. Taste and, if needed, season with pepper and salt.

Notes: If you have a slow cooker or crockpot, put all ingredients stir to combine, and cook for 3-4 hours on HIGH or for 6-8 hours on LOW.

BLT Filled Avocados
Serves: 8

Prep. Time: 10 minutes

Nutrition Facts per Serving: Calories 580; Total Fat 50.4g; Saturated Fat 11.4g; Cholesterol 24mg; Sodium 589mg; Potassium 1224mg; Total Carbohydrates 25.9g; Dietary Fiber 14.3g; Sugars 3.2g; Protein 12.4g; Vitamin A 14%; Vitamin C 45%; and

Calcium 5%; and Iron 13%

Ingredients:

- 1 cup fresh bread cubes (Sourdough or any crusty bread)
- 1 cup romaine lettuce, chopped, loosely packed
- 1 cup tomatoes, chopped
- 2 tablespoons mayonnaise
- 4 ripe avocados, large-sized
- 80 grams Bacon
- Salt and Pepper, to taste

Directions:

1. Heat a skillet on medium heat. Put the bacon in the skillet and cook each side for about 5 minutes or until crispy. Transfer into a plate lined with paper towel. Add the bread cubes into the bacon fat and cook for about 5 minutes or until the bread cubes are crispy and brown.
2. Chop the crisp bacon into small-sized pieces and put into a bowl. Add the croutons, romaine, and tomatoes. Add the mayonnaise and stir to coat. Season with salt and pepper to taste.
3. Slice the avocado into halves. Remove the seed and the pit. Sprinkle the tops with salt.
4. Divide the BLT mixture between each avocado, spooning into the avocado wells. Serve!

Avocado Chicken Lime Soup
Serves: 6

Prep. Time: 15 minutes

Cook Time: 20 minutes

Nutrition Facts per Serving: Calories 386; Total Fat 25.3g; Saturated Fat 5.2g;

Cholesterol 25mg; Sodium 202mg; Potassium 804mg; Total Carbohydrates 30.1g; Dietary Fiber 10.3g; Sugars 2.6g; Protein 13.9g; Vitamin A 17%; Vitamin C 37%; Calcium 7%; and Iron 12%

Ingredients::

- 8 ounces tortilla chips, for serving
- 4 cans (14.5 ounces) chicken broth, low-sodium
- 3 tablespoons fresh squeezed lime juice
- 3 avocados, medium-sized, peeled, cored, and then diced
- 2 Roma tomatoes, seeded and then diced
- 2 jalapeno peppers, seeds removed and then minced
- 2 cloves garlic, minced

- 170 grams chicken breasts, boneless, skinless
- 1/3 cup cilantro, chopped
- 1/2 teaspoon ground cumin
- 1 tablespoon olive oil
- 1 cup green onions, chopped (including whites, white parts minced)
- Salt and fresh ground black pepper

Directions:

1. Put 1 tablespoon oil in a large-sized pot and heat on medium heat. When hot, add the jalapeno and green onions; sauté for about 2 minutes or until tender. Add the garlic during the last 30 seconds of sautéing the green onions and jalapeno.
2. Pour the chicken broth into the pot. Add the cumin, tomatoes, and season to taste with pepper and salt. Add the chicken and bring to a boil on medium-high heat. When boiling, reduce the heat to medium. Cover the pot with lid and cook, occasionally stirring, for about 10-15 minutes or until the chicken is cooked.
3. Reduce the heat to very low and transfer the chicken onto a cutting board. Let rest for 5 minutes and then shred into pieces. Return the shredded chicken into the soup. Stir in the lime juice and cilantro.
4. Just before serving, add the avocados. If not serving right away, then just add the

avocados into each serving bowl, about 1/2 avocado per serving.

5. Serve with tortillas.

Green Pea Guacamole Lettuce or Kale Wraps

Serves: 2

Prep. Time: 10 minutes

Nutrition Facts per Serving: Calories 298; Total Fat 20.4g; Saturated Fat 4.3g;

Cholesterol 12mg; Sodium 138mg; Potassium 755mg; Total Carbohydrates 22.1g; Dietary Fiber 11.0g; Sugars 5.7g; Protein 10.5g; Vitamin A 18%; Vitamin C 78%; Calcium 4%; and Iron 11%

Ingredients:

- 1 cup green peas, steamed or fresh
- 1 lime, juice only
- 1 small-sized avocado or 1/2 large-sized
- 1/4 cup fresh cilantro leaves, chopped
- 1/4-1/2 jalapeño pepper, chopped, optional
- 3 chives OR 1/4 cup red onion, chopped
- 30 grams cooked chicken, shredded
- Kale OR lettuce, to wrap
- Sea salt, if desired

Directions:

1. Put the avocado, peas, cilantro, and lime juice into a food processor. Process until well incorporated, stopping and scrapping the sides down of the food processor as needed.
2. Transfer the mixture into a bowl.
3. Add the chives or onion, jalapeno pepper, and, if using, salt to taste.
4. Add the shredded chicken and tomatoes and stir to combine.
5. Scoop the mixture into large pieces of leafy green leaves of your choice. Enjoy.

Tomato and Avocado Salad
Serves: 2

Prep. Time: 10 minutes

Nutrition Facts per Serving: Calories 507; Total Fat 40.5g; Saturated Fat 8.5g;

Cholesterol 23mg8; Sodium 118mg; Potassium 1441mg; Total Carbohydrates 29.6g;

Dietary Fiber 16.3g; Sugars 7.1g; Protein 14.3g; Vitamin A 28%; Vitamin C 83%; Calcium 6%; and Iron 11%

Ingredients:

- 60 grams cooked chicken, shredded OR 60 grams canned tuna, drained
- 2 tomatoes, large-sized, cut into large-sized dices
- 2 tablespoons cilantro, chopped
- 2 limes, juice only
- 2 avocados, cut into large-sized dice
- 1 red onion, small-sized, thinly sliced
- Extra-virgin olive oil
- Salt

Directions:

1. In a large-sized bowl, combine the avocado, tomato, cilantro, and red onions. Squeeze the lime juice and drizzle the olive oil over the top. Stir gently. Taste and season with salt, as desired.
2. Divide into 2 servings. Divide the chicken/tuna between each serving, topping the meat on top of each. Serve.

Panzanella Lunch
Serves: 2

Prep. Time: 20 minutes

Nutrition Facts per Serving: Calories 223; Total Fat 8.3g; Saturated Fat 2.0g;

Cholesterol 14mg; Sodium 236mg; Potassium 620mg; Total Carbohydrates 25.3g; Dietary Fiber 3.7g; Sugars 8.6g; Protein 12.3g; Vitamin A 29%; Vitamin C 43%; Calcium 9%; and Iron 12%

Ingredients:

- 1 1/2 cups cucumber, coarsely chopped
- 1 1/2 teaspoons extra-virgin olive oil
- 1 tablespoon red wine vinegar
- 1/2 cup red onion, thinly sliced
- 1/2 ounce (about 1/2 Tablespoon) feta cheese
- 2 ounces country bread, thick-sliced, toasted
- 50 grams tuna
- 8 ounces tomatoes, vine-ripened, coarsely chopped (about 1 1/2 cups)
- Fresh ground black pepper

Directions:

1. Slice the toasted bread into 1-inch cubes, making about 2 cups and then transfer into a portable container.
2. Add the feta cheese, tomatoes, red onion, and cucumber. Lightly toss and then sprinkle with the olive oil, rice vinegar, and pepper to taste. Lightly toss again.
3. The salad is marinated at its best when the tomato juices have soaked into the bread cubes.
4. Keep for up to 3 hours at room temperature or for up to 6 hours in the refrigerator.

Deviled Egg Finger Sandwiches
Serves: 2

Prep. Time: 10 minutes

Nutrition Facts per Serving: Calories 304; Total Fat 14.6g; Saturated Fat 3.6g;

Cholesterol 331mg; Sodium 366mg; Potassium 457mg; Total Carbohydrates 29.9g; Dietary Fiber 0.9g; Sugars 15.7g; Protein 13.7g; Vitamin A 12%; Vitamin C 216%; Calcium 8%; and Iron 24%

Ingredients:

- 1 1/2 teaspoon apple cider vinegar
- 1/2 teaspoon Worcestershire sauce
- 1/4 teaspoon paprika
- 2 tablespoons mayonnaisc
- 4 eggs, large-sized, hard-boiled, egg yolks and egg whites separated
- 4 slices white bread
- Paprika and chives, for garnishing
- Salt and pepper, to taste
- 1 1/4 cups fresh squeezed orange juice, divided into 2 servings

Directions:

1. Put the egg yolks into a medium-sized bowl. Add the Worcestershire sauce, mayonnaise, vinegar, and paprika, and mash using a fork – mix until smooth. If needed, add more mayonnaise for a creamy, smooth texture.
2. Dice the egg whites into fine pieces and add into the egg yolk mixture. Season with pepper and salt to taste.
3. Divide the egg salad into2 portions and sandwich between slices of bread. Slice the bread into triangles. If desired, sprinkle the top of the sandwiches with paprika. Serve.

Notes: You can hard boil the eggs a couple of days ahead. The egg salad can also be made ahead of time –keep covered in the refrigerator until assembling the sandwich.

Zoodle French Onion Bake
Serves: 4

Prep. Time: 15 minutes

Cook Time: 40 minutes

Nutrition Facts per Serving: Calories 259; Total Fat 15.3g; Saturated Fat 9.1g; Cholesterol 47mg; Sodium 524mg; Potassium 287mg; Total Carbohydrates 20.8g;

Dietary Fiber 2.1g; Sugars 5.5g; Protein 10.5g; Vitamin A 12%; Vitamin C 23%; Calcium 21%; and Iron 10%

Ingredients:

- 1 cup fontina cheese, grated
- 1 teaspoon fresh thyme, chopped (PLUS more for garnish)
- 1 teaspoon granulated sugar
- 1 yellow onion, small-sized, sliced thinly
- 1/4 cup beef broth
- 2 1/2 cups zucchini noodles (or two medium sized zucchinis)
- 2 tablespoons unsalted butter
- 2 teaspoons Worcestershire sauce
- 3 slices toasted bread, per serving

- Salt and pepper to taste

Directions:

1. Preheat the oven to 400F.
2. Heat a skillet over medium heat. Add the butter and the onion. Sauté for a few minutes. Add the Worcestershire sauce, sugar, pepper, salt, and thyme. Stir and cook for a few minutes more. Add the beef broth and cook for about 12 minutes or until the onion is golden brown, occasionally stirring to prevent the onion from burning.
3. Grease a 8x5-inch baking dish with nonstick cooking spray.
4. In a large-sized bowl, combine the French onion and the zoodles. Pour the mixture into the greased dish, spreading in an even layer. Top with the Fontina cheese.
5. Put the baking dish in the oven and bake for about 20-25 minutes or until golden brown.
6. Remove the baking dish from the oven and let the bake slightly cool before serving.

If desired, garnish with fresh thyme. Liquid may appear from the zucchini. If this happens, carefully drain off using a spoon before serving.

SNACK RECIPES

Cauliflower Hash Browns
Serves: 2

Prep. Time: 30 min

Cook Time: 15 min

Nutrition Facts per Serving: Calories 279;
Total Fat 12.1g; Saturated Fat 6.8g; Cholesterol
112mg37%; Sodium 829mg35%; Potassium
903mg26%; Total Carbohydrates 30.7g;
Dietary Fiber 3.9g; Sugars 21.8g; Protein 14.0g;
Vitamin A 8%; Vitamin C 405%; Calcium 25%;
and Iron 22%

Ingredients:

- 1 egg, large-sized
- 1 small-sized head cauliflower, grated
- 1/2 cup Cheddar Cheese, Shredded
- 1/2 teaspoon black pepper
- 1/2 teaspoon Cayenne Pepper, optional
- 1/2 teaspoon salt
- 1/4 teaspoon garlic powder
- 1 3/4 cups fresh squeezed orange juice, divided into 2 servings

Directions:

1. Grate the whole cauliflower head.
2. Put in microwavable bowl and microwave for 3 minutes and then let cool. When cool, put in a cheesecloth or paper towel and squeeze out all excess moisture.
3. Put the squeezed dried cauliflower into a large-sized bowl. Add the rest of the ingredients and then combine until well mixed.
4. Form the cauliflower mixture into 6 pieces square-shaped hash browns on a greased baking tray.
5. Put the baking tray in a preheated 400F oven and bake for about 15-20 minutes.
6. Remove the baking tray from the oven. Let the hash cool for 10 minutes to firm up. Serve while still warm.

Honey Drizzled Pistachio and Avocado Bagel Toast
Serves: 1

Prep. Time: 5 minutes

Nutrition Facts per Serving: Calories 384; Total Fat 24.9g; Saturated Fat 7.7g; Cholesterol 36mg; Sodium 700mg; Potassium 449mg; Total Carbohydrates 28.9g; Dietary Fiber 4.4g; Sugars 10.6g; Protein 13.7g; Vitamin A 4%; Vitamin C 9%; Calcium 5%; and Iron 15%

Ingredients:

- 1 bagel (your favorite flavor), sliced into 2 round halves
- 1/2 ripe avocado, sliced
- 2 tablespoons cream cheese, softened
- 2 tablespoons pistachios, chopped
- 3 teaspoons honey
- 45 grams bacon, cooked and crumbled
- Ground black pepper and sea salt

Directions:

1. Toast the bagel to your desired crispness. With the cut side faced put, put the roasted bagels halves into a plate. Spread each cut top with 1 tablespoon cream cheese and then top with avocado slices.
2. Sprinkle with the pistachios and then with pepper and salt to taste.
3. Drizzle each with honey. Enjoy!

Cauliflower-Gruyere Flatbread

Serves: 4

Prep. Time: 10 min

Cook Time: 5 min

Nutrition Facts per Serving: Calories 286; Total Fat 12.7g; Saturated Fat 7.2g; Cholesterol 41mg; Sodium 221mg; Potassium 638mg; Total Carbohydrates 30.3g; Dietary Fiber 3.0g; Sugars 15.4g; Protein 14.2g; Vitamin A 8%; Vitamin C 282%; Calcium 38%; Iron 19%

Ingredients:

- 4 1/2 ounces gruyere, grated
- 2 teaspoons fresh thyme leaves
- 1/4 cup half-and-half
- 1 small-sized head cauliflower (about 3/4 pound), cored
- 1 piece naan bread
- 1 clove garlic, minced2 1/2 cups fresh squeezed orange juice, divided into 4 servings

Directions:

1. Preheat the oven to broil.
2. Put 1/2 head of the cauliflower and garlic into a food processor; pulse until resembling fine crumbs.
3. Stir half-and-half in the cauliflower-garlic mixture and season with pepper and salt to taste.
4. Evenly spread the cauliflower the mixture over the naan bread. Separate the remaining 1/2 head cauliflower into small-sized florets and evenly sprinkle on the naan. Top with the grated gruyere.
5. Broil in the oven for about 5 minutes or until the cheese is melted. Sprinkle with thyme and then cut the bread into slices. Serve.

Pepperoni Pizza Pretzels
Serves: 6

Prep. Time: 30 minutes

Cook Time: 20 minutes

Nutrition Facts per Serving: Calories 524; Total Fat 39.3g; Saturated Fat 13.8g; Trans Fat 0.5g; Cholesterol 50mg; Sodium 902mg; Potassium 120mg; Total Carbohydrates 27.8g; Dietary Fiber 2.2g; Protein 13.1g; Vitamin A 5%; Vitamin C 0%; Calcium 10%; and Iron 12%

Ingredients:

- 1 can pizza dough
- 1/2 teaspoon garlic, minced
- 1/2 teaspoon Italian seasoning
- 1/4 cup parmesan, shredded
- 170 grams mini pepperonis OR normal-sized pepperonis sliced into pieces
- 2 tablespoons butter, melted
- 60 grams Italian cheese, shredded

Directions:

1. Preheat the oven to 400F.
2. Open and unroll the pizza dough. Along the shorter side, slice the dough into 6 pieces.
3. Evenly divide and sprinkle the pepperonis onto slice of dough. Horizontally fold each dough over so that the edges meet and then pinch along where they meet so the pepperonis and cheese are inside.
4. Twist the folded dough into pretzel shapes by crossing the dough ad twisting around where it crosses. Put the ends of the dough near the middle, creating a bit of space in between.
5. In a small-sized bowl, combine the melted butter with the minced garlic and Italian seasoning. Drizzle the mixture over the top of each pretzel.
6. Line a cookie sheet with parchment paper and then arrange the pretzels in the cookie sheet.
7. Put the cookie sheet in the oven and bake for about 20 minutes or until the pretzels are slightly browned.
8. When baked, pull the pretzels off the parchment paper. Let cool for a bit and serve.

Streusel Topped Whole-Wheat Cranberry Apple Muffins
Serves: 12

Prep. Time: 10 minutes

Cook Time: 18-20 minutes

Nutrition Facts per Serving: Calories 336; Total Fat 21.1g; Saturated Fat 6.7g; Trans Fat 0.1g; Cholesterol 49mg; Sodium 492mg; Potassium 228mg; Total Carbohydrates 24.4g; Dietary Fiber 0.6g; Sugars 14.4g; Protein 12.0g; Vitamin A 2%; Vitamin C 1%; Calcium 5%; and Iron 8%

Ingredients:

- 4 links sausages per serving, cooked, for serving

For the dry ingredients:

- 1 cup whole-wheat flour
- 1 teaspoon cinnamon
- 1/2 teaspoon baking powder
- 1/4 teaspoon allspice
- 1/4 teaspoon nutmeg
- 3/4 teaspoon baking soda

For the wet ingredients:

- 1 medium-sized apple, peeled and finely chopped
- 1 teaspoon vanilla extract
- 1/2 cup yogurt
- 1/3 cup honey
- 1/4 cup dried cranberries, roughly chopped
- 1/4 cup olive oil or canola oil

For the streusel ingredients:

- 1 1/2 teaspoon cinnamon
- 1/2 cup brown sugar
- 2 tablespoons butter, melted
- 3 tablespoons wheat flour

Directions:

1. Combine all he dry ingredients in a bowl and set aside.
2. In a large-sized bowl, whisk together all the wet ingredients until smooth and well combined.
3. Add the dry ingredients into the bowl of wet ingredients and mix gently to combine – do not beat or the muffins will come out hard, just combine.

4. Preheat the oven to 350F. Line 12 muffin cups with liners and gently grease the liners with cooking spray.
5. In a bowl, combined all the streusel ingredients and keep ready.
6. Scoop the batter into each lined muffin cup, filling each 3/4 full.
7. Divide and sprinkle the streusel on top of each muffin.
8. Bake for about 18-20 minutes or until a toothpick comes out clean when inserted in the center of the muffins.
9. Remove the muffins from the oven and let rest in the cups for about 5 minutes. Gently take them out and put on a wire rack to cool completely.
10. Store the muffins in airtight containers.

Cheese and Bacon Egg McMuffin-Copy-Cat Cups
Serves: 6

Prep. Time: 25 minutes

Cook Time: 15-20 minutes

Nutrition Facts per Serving: Calories 275; Total Fat 10.9g; Saturated Fat 4.5g; Cholesterol 181mg; Sodium 389mg; Potassium 466mg; Total Carbohydrates 30.3g; Dietary Fiber 1.3g; Sugars 15.3g; Protein 13.9g; Vitamin A 6%; Vitamin C 231%; Calcium 14%; Iron 23%

Ingredients:

- 6 slices bacon, ready cooked - not microwaved, just right out of the package
- 6 eggs, large-sized
- 3 whole English muffins, split into top and bottom halves
- 1/2 cup cheddar cheese, shredded
- Pinches fresh ground black pepper
- Pinches kosher salt
- 4 cups orange juice, divided into 6 servings

Directions:

1. Preheat the oven to 350F. Press an English muffin half carefully into the bottom of a Texas-sized muffin cup tin Form a bacon piece into a small circle and put on the inside of the muffin. Repeat the process with the remaining muffin halves and bacons.
2. Divide the cheese into 6 portions and sprinkle each portion on the muffin inside the bacon ring.
3. Crack and break an egg inside the bacon ring, making sure the egg yolks stay intact. Sprinkle the eggs with pinches of salt and pepper.
4. Bake for about 15-20 minutes or until the eggs are cooked through and not jiggly.
5. Remove the muffin tin from the oven and let the muffins cool for 5 minutes before removing them. Serve.

Fried Provolone, Crumbled Bacon, and Tomato Sandwich
Serves: 2

Nutrition Facts per Serving: Calories 297; Total Fat 19.1g; Saturated Fat 6.7g; Cholesterol 30mg; Sodium 641mg; Potassium 366mg; Total Carbohydrates 21.6g; Dietary Fiber 1.9g; Sugars 6.1g; Protein 10.8g; Vitamin A 27%; Vitamin C 28%; Calcium 26%; and Iron 7%

Ingredients:

- 2 tomatoes, medium-sized, perfectly ripe, sliced
- 2-4 slices (1/4-inch) provolone cheese (use larger amount for smaller slices)
- 4 slices (1/2-inch thick) your favorite sturdy bread
- 4 tablespoons mayonnaise
- 5 grams bacon, cooked, crumbled
- Flaky salt, to taste
- Fresh ground black pepper, to taste
- Olive oil

Directions:

1. Spread 1 tablespoon mayonnaise on one side of each bread and set aside.
2. Heat a nonstick skillet on medium-low heat. Put a thin layer of oil in the skillet and heat until shimmering. Add 1 slice of provolone cheese in the skillet and fry until the bottom is golden and crusty. With a very thin spatula, carefully lift and flip the cheese – it will probably not flip neatly, but a messy cheese slice will still be as delicious. Fry until the other side is golden and crusty. Lift the cheese from the skillet and put on a prepared slice of bread. Repeat the process with the remaining cheese – you can cook more than 1 cheese at a time if you are comfortable with it.
3. Divide and sprinkle the crumbled bacon over the cheese. Divide and arrange the slices of tomatoes on top and sprinkle with pepper and salt. Top with the remaining slice of bread. Serve.

Crusty Herb-Parmesan Zucchini Bites
Serves: 4

Prep. Time: 20 minutes

Cook Time: 15 minutes

Nutrition Facts per Serving: Calories 111; Total Fat 3.8g; Saturated Fat 2.3g; Cholesterol 11mg; Sodium 160mg; Potassium 631mg; Total Carbohydrates 14.8g; Dietary Fiber 4.2g; Sugars 8.8g; Protein 7.8g; Vitamin A 14%; Vitamin C 108%; Calcium 21%; and Iron 10%

Ingredients:

- 60 grams fresh Parmesan cheese, grated
- 4 fresh zucchini, medium-sized, sliced lengthwise in halves
- 1-2 tablespoons fresh rosemary and thyme, minced
- Salt and pepper, to taste
- Smidge olive oil
- 1 1/4 orange, peeled, wedges separated, divide wedges into 4 servings

Directions:

1. Preheat the oven to 350F.
2. Lightly brush both sides of the zucchini with olive oil and put into a baking sheet lined with aluminum foil.
3. In a small-sized bowl, mix the herbs and the cheese together and then sprinkle over the zucchini and then sprinkle with pepper and salt.
4. Bake in the oven for 15 minutes and then broil for the last 3 to 5 minutes or until the cheese is brown and crispy.

Roasted Asparagus with Shallot Mustard Sauce
Serves: 2

Prep. Time: 10 minutes

Cook Time: 10 minutes

Nutrition Facts per Serving: Calories 405; Total Fat 33.2g; Saturated Fat 15.7g; Cholesterol 4mg; Sodium 133mg; Potassium 841mg; Total Carbohydrates 23.5g; Dietary Fiber 8.9g; Sugars 11.4g; Protein 11.4g; Vitamin A 40%; Vitamin C 67%; Calcium 18%; and Iron 42%

Ingredients:

For the asparagus:

- 1 bunch (1 pound) asparagus
- 1/2 cup coconut milk
- 1/2 teaspoon dried thyme
- 1/4-1/2 cup chicken broth
- 2 shallot bulbs, medium-sized, sliced thin
- 2 tablespoons mustard - spicy, whole grain, or 'deli-style'
- 2 tablespoons olive or coconut oil, divided

- Salt and pepper, to taste
- 1/2 orange, peeled, wedges separated divided into 2 portions
- Cheese, divided into 2 portions

Directions:

For the asparagus:

1. Wash the asparagus clean and then snap off the woody end portions.
2. Set an oven rack in the middle position and preheat the broiler on HIGH.
3. When the asparagus is dry, put in a rimmed baking sheet, arranging them in a single layer. Drizzle with 1 tablespoon oil and season to taste with salt and pepper. Toss to distribute the spices and oil.
4. Put the baking sheet in the race and broil for 4 minutes. After 4 minutes, roll each asparagus halfway using a pair of tongs so the previous bottom sides are facing up.
5. Broil for 4-6 minutes more or until some spots of the asparagus become dark – do not let them burn.
6. Remove the baking sheet from the oven. Transfer the asparagus onto a serving platter or onto individual plates.

For the sauce:

1. Put 1 tablespoon oil into a skillet and heat over medium heat. When the oil is shimmering hot, add the shallots and stir to coat with oil. Reduce the heat to medium-low. Cook the shallots, occasionally stirring, until soft and translucent, but not dark and crispy.
2. Add the chicken broth and the coconut milk. With a nylon spatula, scrape the bottom of the skillet to remove any delicious browned bits stuck in the bottom and stir thoroughly to combine.
3. Add the mustard and stir until completely combined and no mustard clump remains. Add the dried thyme and quickly stir it in. Bring the sauce to a simmer, occasionally stirring and scraping the bottom of the skillet to prevent from burning.
4. When the sauce reaches desired thickness, remove from the heat. Pour the sauce over the roasted cauliflower and serve. Enjoy with wedges of orange on the side.

Jalapeno Meatball Ring
Serves: 8

Prep. Time: 20 minutes

Cook Time: 20 minutes

Nutrition Facts per Serving: Calories 252; Total Fat 9.8g; Saturated Fat 3.3g; Cholesterol 21mg; Sodium 473mg; Potassium 195mg; Total Carbohydrates 29.9g; Dietary Fiber 2.3g; Sugars 4.8g; Protein 14.2g; Vitamin A 9%; Vitamin C 15%;

Calcium 9%; and Iron 10%

Ingredients:

- 1 cup mozzarella cheese, shredded
- 1/2 white onion, diced
- 12 ounces meatballs (I used Farm Rich Original Meatball)
- 13 ounces canned crescent roll dough
- 3 jalapeno peppers, sliced
- 3 Roma tomatoes, chopped
- 6 slices provolone cheese, divided in half

Directions:

1. Preheat the oven to 375F.
2. Use a nonstick cookie sheet or line a regular cookie sheet with parchment paper.
3. Prepare the meatballs following the directions of the microwave. Cut the meatballs into halves and set aside.
4. Unroll the crescent roll dough and separate 13 ounces into triangles (save the excess triangles). Arrange the triangles in the cookie sheet into a circle, overlapping the edges.
5. Top with the cheese, meatballs, tomatoes, mozzarella cheese, jalapeno peppers, and onions.
6. Put the cookie sheet in the oven. Bake for about 15 to 20 minutes or until golden brown.
7. Let the meatball ring cool for 2 minutes before slicing. Enjoy!

Crunchy Crescent Havarti and Ham
Serves: 20

Prep. Time: 10 minutes

Cook Time: 20 minutes

Nutrition Facts per Serving: Calories 162; Total Fat 6.6g; Saturated Fat 2.8g; Cholesterol 28mg; Sodium 438mg; Potassium 100mg; Total Carbohydrates 17.1g; Dietary Fiber 1.0g; Sugars 2.3g; Protein 8.6g; Vitamin A 2%; Vitamin C 1%; Calcium 12%; and Iron 8%

Ingredients:

- 6 slices Havarti cheese
- 20 ounces crescent roll dough, without perforations, store-bought
- 2 tablespoons all-purpose flour
- 12 ounces ham slices
- 1 tablespoon water
- 1 egg, beaten
- 1 1/2 teaspoons poppy seeds
- 1 1/2 teaspoons dehydrated onions
- 1 1/2 tablespoons sweet pickle relish
- 1 1/2 tablespoons mustard, deli-style

Directions:

1. Preheat the oven to 400F.
2. On a nonstick baking sheet, unroll and flatten 10-ounce worth crescent dough into an even rectangle (save the excess dough for other recipes).
3. Evenly top the dough with the slices of ham, leaving a 1/4-inch border around the edges.
4. Evenly top the ham slices with pickle relish, mustard, and cheese.
5. On a lightly floured work surface, unroll and flatten another 10-ounce worth crescent dough and flatten into the same size as the first dough. Carefully transfer the dough, placing it over the top of the other dough to cover the filling. With a fork, press all the 4 edges to seal and then with a paring knife, cut 3 small-sized steam holes in the top dough (save the excess dough for other recipes).
6. Mix the water and egg. Brush the top of the dough with the egg wash. Sprinkle the top of the dough with dehydrated onion and poppy seeds.
7. Bake in the oven for about 20 to 25 minutes or until the dough is golden brown.
8. Remove from the oven, let slightly cool, slice, and serve while still warm.

Cheesy Spinach Pinwheels

Serves: 24 pinwheels (3 pinwheels per serving)

Prep. Time: 35 minutes

Cook Time: 20 minutes

Nutrition Facts per Serving: Calories 139; Total Fat 4.9g; Saturated Fat 1.9g; Cholesterol 16mg; Sodium 501mg; Potassium 195mg; Total Carbohydrates 16.2g; Dietary Fiber 1.0g; Sugars 2.4g; Protein 8.2g; Vitamin A 41%; Vitamin C 10%; Calcium 9%; and Iron 9%

Ingredients:

- 1 1/2 ounces Parmesan cheese, freshly and finely grated (shred on the smallest box grater hole)
- 1 ounce feta cheese, crumbled
- 1 sheet (about 249 grams) frozen puff pastry, defrosted (such as Pepperidge Farms)
- 2 garlic cloves, minced
- 2 teaspoons olive oil
- 6 ounces fresh spinach, torn or chopped into pieces
- 90 grams cooked chicken, shredded
- Salt and pepper, to taste

Directions:

1. Sprinkle a little flour on a dry, clean work area –this will prevent the pastry from sticking. Put the puff pastry on the floured surface ad with a rolling pin, roll the pastry into a 14x10-inch even rectangle.
2. Put the olive oil in a large-sized sauté pan or skillet and heat over medium heat. Add the garlic and cook for 1 minute. Add the spinach, stir to mix, and cook for about 2 to 3 minutes, stirring occasionally, until wilted. Season with a few shakes of pepper and salt to taste.
3. Evenly spread the spinach mixture across the surface of the pastry, covering the entire surface.
4. With the longer side of the pastry rectangle facing you, roll by pushing forward, wrapping the ingredients, and creating a long roll or a big log. Wrap the roll. Log with a cling wrap or a parchment paper and freeze for about 30 to 40 minutes – this will make it easier to cut the roll/log into circles.
5. Preheat the oven to 400F. Line a large-sized baking sheet with parchment paper and set aside.
6. Take the pastry roll/log out from the freezer. With a serrated knife, slice the roll/log into 24 spirals – slice the roll/log in half, then each half into quarters, and then cut the quarters into thirds.

7. Put the pinwheels in the prepared baking sheet and bake for about 20 minutes or until lightly golden. Serve while still warm.

Jalapeno Poppers

Serves: 24 popper (2 poppers per serving)

Prep. Time: 10 minutes

Cook Time: 20 minutes

Nutrition Facts per Serving: Calories 242; Total Fat 15.4g; Saturated Fat 9.6g; Cholesterol 49mg; Sodium 1015mg; Potassium 378mg; Total Carbohydrates 18.9g; Dietary Fiber 4.3g; Sugars 13.8g; Protein 9.2g; Vitamin A 32%; Vitamin C 124%; Calcium 26%; and Iron 8%

Ingredients:

- 12 jalapeno peppers, large-sized
- 2 ounces feta cheese
- 4 ounces cream cheese, at room temperature
- 4 ounces sharp cheddar cheese, shredded
- 1 teaspoon onion powder, or more to taste
- 1 small handful fresh cilantro, finely chopped
- 4 1/4 orange, peeled, wedges separated, divided into 6 portions

Directions:

1. Preheat the oven to 425F.
2. In a lengthwise manner, slice the jalapeno peppers into halves and scoop out the seeds and the insides.
3. Put the cream cheese, feta cheese, cheddar cheese, onion powder, and cilantro in a bowl and mash until well mixed.
4. Divide the cheese mixture between the jalapeno, filling them up.
5. Roast for about 15 to 20 minutes or until the jalapeno peppers are tender and the edges of the cheese stuffing is brown and bubbly.

Chipotle Meatballs

Serves: 24 balls (2 balls per serving)

Prep. Time: 30 minutes

Cook Time: 6-10 minutes

Nutrition Facts per Serving: Calories 164; Total Fat 9.1g; Saturated Fat 2.9g; Cholesterol 13mg; Sodium 349mg; Potassium 135mg; Total Carbohydrates 14.6g; Dietary Fiber 1.8g; Sugars 2.8g; Protein 7.3g; Vitamin A 2%; Vitamin C 19%; Calcium 11%; and Iron 5%

Ingredients:

- 1 avocado, medium-sized, pitted, and then peeled, cut into 24 small-sized slices
- 1 can refrigerated crescent dinner rolls (I used Pillsbury™)
- 1 chipotles in adobo sauce, finely chopped PLUS 3 tablespoons adobo sauce
- 1 tablespoon vegetable oil
- 1/2 cups onion, finely chopped
- 12 frozen Italian-style meatballs, 1/2 ounce each, thawed and halved
- 4 pieces (1 ounces each) mozzarella string cheese

Directions:

1. Preheat the oven to 350F. Grease a 24-cup mini muffin tin with nonstick cooking spray.
2. Separate the dough into 4 rectangles. Press the perforations to seal and then slice each rectangle into 6 squares.
3. Press each square into the bottom and up the sides of each mini muffin cup. Bake for 6 minutes in the oven. With the handle of a wooden spoon, immediately create a 1 1/2-inch indentation in the center of each cup.
4. Meanwhile, put the oil in a 10-inch skillet and heat on medium heat. Add the onion and cook for about 2 to 3 minutes or until softened. Stir in the chipotle pepper and the adobo sauce. Add the meatballs and 2 tablespoons water. Cover the skillet and reduce the heat to low. Cook for about 3-4 minutes, occasionally stirring or until heated thoroughly. Remove the meatballs from the skillet. Spoon 1/2 teaspoon of the sauce into each indentation of the cups and then top each with 1 meatball half, placing the meatball half with the cut side faced up.
5. Slice each mozzarella cheese lengthwise into halves and then cut each half crosswise into thirds. Top each meatball with 1 piece mozzarella cheese. Bake for about 6-10

minutes or until the edges of the pastry are golden brown. Let cool for 1 minute before removing from the cups.

Top each meatball cup with 1 slice avocado and secure with a wooden toothpick, piercing each cup in the center. Serve warm

DINNER RECIPES

Sautéed Vegetables and Salmon
Serves: 4

Prep. Time: 5 minutes

Cook Time: 15 minutes

Nutrition Facts per Serving: Calories 140; Total Fat 5.0g; Saturated Fat 3.2g; Cholesterol 9mg; Sodium 86mg; Potassium 685mg; Total Carbohydrates 17.0g; Dietary Fiber 5.5g; Sugars 8.1g; Protein 8.5g; Vitamin A 307%; Vitamin C 140%; Calcium 9%; and Iron 13%

Ingredients:

- 3/4 pounds carrots
- 2 cups snow peas
- 2 cups broccoli florets
- 1 tablespoon coconut oil
- Salt and pepper
- 80 grams cooked salmon

Directions:

1. Under cold water, rinse the broccoli and snow peas to remove any dirt.
2. Peel the carrots and then slice them into thin round, or, if they are very large, cut into halves and slice the halves into thin half moons.
3. Heat a large-sized pan on medium-high heat, add the oil, and melt. Add he vegetables and stir to coat with oil; sauté for about 5 minutes, occasionally stirring.
4. When the veggies start to slightly brown, reduce the heat to low or medium and cover the pan with a lid. Cook for about 5 to 10 minutes or until the carrots are soft, but can still hold their shape.
5. When the veggies are cooked, season with salt and pepper. Divide the sautéed veggies between 4 serving bowl. Divide the cooked salmon between each bowl, topping them on the veggies. Serve!

Roasted Cauliflower Salad with Maple-Balsamic Reduction

Serves: 6

Prep. Time: 10 minutes

Cook Time: 25 minutes

Nutrition Facts per Serving: Calories 201; Total Fat 3.7g; Saturated Fat 0.6g; Cholesterol 21mg; Sodium 93mg; Potassium 682mg; Total Carbohydrates 30.6g; Dietary Fiber 6.3g; Sugars 10.5g; Protein 14.1g; Vitamin A 9%; Vitamin C 120%;

Calcium 7%; Iron 13%

Ingredients

For the salad:

- 1 cauliflower, large-sized
- 1 cup roast buckwheat
- 1 large handful parsley, chopped finely
- 1/2 pomegranate seeds
- 1/2 teaspoon ground cinnamon
- 1/2 teaspoon ground cumin
- 1/4 teaspoon ground coriander
- 1/8 teaspoon chili powder

- 2 handfuls slivered almonds, roasted in a dry pan
- 160 grams cooked chicken, shredded OR 160 grams canned tuna, drained
- Olive oil
- Salt

For the reduction:

- 3 tablespoons (45 ml) maple syrup
- 6 tablespoons (90 ml) balsamic vinegar

Directions:

1. Preheat the oven to 430F or 220C. Line a baking tray with 1 piece of baking paper.
2. In a small-sized bowl, combine all the spices and 1/4 teaspoon fine sea salt.
3. Cut the cauliflower into large-sized florets, coat with olive oil, and then sprinkle with the prepared spice mixture.
4. Transfer the seasoned cauliflower florets into the prepared baking tray; bake for about 25 minutes or until cooked and charred nicely charred in some places.
5. Carefully pick the buckwheat, removing any debris and small stones – do not rinse, otherwise it will become mushy.
6. Put the buckwheat into a small-sized pot with a glass lid. Add 1 1/2 cups or 360 ml water into the pot. Cover the pot with the lid and bring to a boil - do not salt until

cooked; salt affects the texture of buckwheat negatively. When the water starts to boil, reduce the heat to low. Cook until the buckwheat absorbs the water – to check, tip the pot to see if water is still coming out from underneath the buckwheat; DO NOT lift the lid to check. When the buckwheat fully absorbs the water, turn the heat off and remove the pot from the heat. Let the pot rest for 10 minutes – make sure the lid is firmly on – to let the buckwheat finish cooking in its own steam. When ready, salt the buckwheat to taste.

7. Put the maple syrup and the balsamic vinegar into a small-sized pot; bring to a boil. When boiling, reduce the heat to low and simmer until reduced by 1/3 and reaches the consistency of a very runny honey – the reduction will thicken as it cools down. If the reduction turns too sticky when it cools down, add 1 splash water into the pot, and return on the stove over ow heat. Immediately remove from the heat when it becomes a homogeneous sauce.

8. In a large bowl, combine the roasted cauliflower and seasoned buckwheat. Generously sprinkle with pomegranate seeds, chopped parsley, roasted slivers of almond, and drizzle with the reduction.

9. Divide the salad between 6 serving bowls. Divide the cooked chicken and top on each serving. Serve.

Broccoli Mac and Cheese
Serves: 8

Prep. Time: 20 minutes

Cook Time: 10 minutes

Nutrition Facts per Serving: Calories 311; Total Fat 16.3g; Saturated Fat 13.1g;

Cholesterol 34mg; Sodium 449mg; Potassium 711mg; Total Carbohydrates 30.4g;

Dietary Fiber 5.1g; Sugars 4.4g; Protein 14.6g; Vitamin A 3%;   Vitamin C 93%; Calcium 5%; and Iron 22%

Ingredients:

For the broccoli mac and cheese:
- 9 1/2 ounces dry short pasta (such as bowties, macaroni, penne, or fusilli)
- 2 cups broccoli (plus stems if you like)
- 100 grams cooked chicken, shredded
- Salt and pepper, to taste

For the cauliflower cream sauce:

- 575 grams cauliflower
- 3 cloves garlic

- 2 teaspoons white miso paste
- 2 cups vegetable broth
- 2 cups non-dairy milk (almond milk or soy milk)
- 1/4 cup nutritional yeast
- 1/2 teaspoon salt, or to taste

Directions:

For the cauliflower cream sauce:

1. Remove the green leaves from the cauliflower and discard. Chop the cauliflower into even-sized pieces – you don't have to cut them into pretty pieces; you will be blending them later. Peel the cloves of garlic and leave them whole.
2. Put the cauliflower in a big pot. Add the vegetable broth, non-dairy milk, and garlic cloves. Bring to a simmer and cook for about 10 minutes or until the cauliflower is very soft and falls apart when pierced with a fork.
3. With an immersion blender, you can blend the cauliflower mixture directly in the pot. Add the white miso paste, nutritional yeast, and salt and blend to mix.
4. Alternatively, you can blend the mixture in batches using a stand mixer – do not fill the blender too high. Otherwise, the hot liquid will explode out from the top. Add the white miso paste, nutritional yeast, and salt and blend to mix.

5. If the sauce is too thin, cook it down for a bit, stirring frequently to prevent it from burning. If the sauce is too thick, add a bit more water or vegetable broth.

For the broccoli mac and cheese:
1. Fill a large pot with water and bring to a boil.
2. Cut the broccoli into florets. Peel the stems and cut them as well. If you do not like broccoli stems, then discard them.
3. Boil the pasta following the directions of the package. When there is only 2 minutes boiling time remaining, add the broccoli to cook along with the pasta.
4. When the pasta and broccoli are cooked, drain and then return into the pot. Stir in the cauliflower cream sauce and season with pepper and salt to taste.
5. Divide the mac and cheese between 8 serving bowls. Divide the chicken and top on each serving. Enjoy!

Vegan Lasagna

Serves: 12

Prep. Time: 35 minutes

Cook Time: 60 minutes

Nutrition Facts per Serving: Calories 271; Total Fat 13.5g; Saturated Fat 2.1g;

Cholesterol 9mg; Sodium 863mg; Potassium 680mg; Total Carbohydrates 28.4g; Dietary Fiber 5.4g; Sugars 6.3g; Protein 13.5g; Vitamin A 28%; Vitamin C 41%; Calcium 20%; and Iron 15%

Ingredients:

For the eggplant:

- 1 1/2 pounds eggplant (about 2 small-sized)
- 1 teaspoon fresh Italian parsley, finely chopped
- 1/2 teaspoon red wine vinegar
- 2 teaspoons kosher salt, plus more as needed
- 4 tablespoons extra-virgin olive oil
- Fresh ground black pepper
- Pinch red pepper flakes

For the sauce:

- 2 tablespoons capers
- 2 garlic cloves, medium-sized, minced
- 2 cans (28-ounce each) whole peeled tomatoes (I used San Marzano)
- 1/4 teaspoon red pepper flakes, plus more as needed
- 1/4 cup extra-virgin olive oil
- 1 yellow onion, medium-sized, finely chopped
- 1 tablespoon tomato paste
- 1 bay leaf
- Kosher salt

For the noodles:

- 12 ounces dried lasagna noodles
- Kosher salt

For the filling:

- 2 1/4 pounds soft tofu, drained
- 1/3 cup Italian parsley leaves, finely chopped
- 1/2 teaspoon fresh ground black pepper, plus more as needed

- 2 tablespoons lemon juice, fresh squeezed, plus more as needed (from about 1/2 lemon)
- 2 teaspoons kosher salt, plus more as needed
- 2 teaspoons lemon zest, finely grated, (from 2 medium-sized lemons)
- 3 tablespoons nutritional yeast, optional

To assemble:

- 1 cup basil leaves, loosely packed (from about 1 bunch), cut into 1/4-inch thick ribbons

Directions:

For the eggplant:

1. Set a rack in the middle of the oven and preheat the oven to 350F.
2. In a lengthwise manner, slice the eggplants into 1/8-inch thick slices. In a single layer, put the eggplant slices flat on the surface of 2 baking sheets, overlapping them slightly, if needed, and then sprinkle them with 1 teaspoon salt.
3. Flip the eggplant slices and then sprinkle again with 1 teaspoon salt; let sit for about 30 minutes or until water beads from the surface. Meanwhile, prepare the sauce.

For the sauce:

1. Fit a food processor with a blade attachment. Put the tomatoes, along with their juices; pulse until coarsely chopped, about 10 pulses – you may need to chop in batches.
2. Put the oil in a large-sized saucepan with a tight-fitting lid and heat over medium-high heat until shimmering. Add the onion and cook; occasionally stirring, for about 3 minutes or until translucent. Add the garlic and cook for about 30 seconds or until fragrant.
3. Push the garlic and onion to one side of the pan. Add the tomato paste into the emptied side of the pan. Slightly cook the paste for about 1-2 minutes to remove the raw flavor, occasionally stirring. Stir the garlic and onion with the paste to combine.
4. Add the chopped tomatoes, red pepper flakes, bay leaf, and a couple pinches of salt. Bring the mixture to a boil. When boiling, reduce the heat to low, cover the pan, and simmer for 45 minutes to infuse the flavors.
5. Add the capers, taste, and if needed, season with extra salt and red pepper flakes. Set aside.

To finish the eggplant:

1. With paper towels, pat both sides of the eggplant slices to dry.

2. Put 1 1/2 teaspoons oil in a nonstick frying pan and heat on medium-high heat. Put just enough eggplant slices to make a single layer in the pan. Sear each side of the eggplant for 2 minutes. Taste, and if needed, season with pepper and salt. Transfer the seared eggplant slices into a plate. Repeat the process with the remaining eggplant slices, adding oil as needed.

3. While the eggplants are cooking, put the remaining 2 tablespoons of olive oil, vinegar, parsley, red pepper flakes, and 1 pinch salt into a large-sized bowl and stir t mix.

4. Transfer the seared slices eggplant into the vinegar-oil mixture; toss to coat. Taste, and if needed, season with extra salt.

For the noodles:

1. Fill a large pot with water and heavily salt it. Bring to a boil on medium-high heat. Add the lasagna noodles and cook for about 7 minutes, occasionally stirring, until al dente. Drain and let cool. When the noodles are cool enough to handle, lay the pieces flat on a lightly greased baking sheet.

For the filling:

1. Put the tofu, lemon zest, parsley, lemon juice, measured pepper and salt, and, if

using, nutritional yeast, in the food processor fitted with a blade attachment; process for about 30seconds or until smooth.

2. Taste and if needed, season with more lemon juice, pepper, and salt. Set aside.

To assemble:

1. Spread a thin layer of tomato sauce into the bottom of a 9x13-inch baking dish.
2. Put a single layer of lasagna noodles on top of the sauce, about 3 regular-sized noodles. Top the noodles with 1/4 of the tofu filling, about 1 cup, and evenly spread. Lay 1/4 of the eggplant slices over the tofu filling and then spread 1 cup sauce over the eggplant. Sprinkle with 1/4 cup basil leaves. Make 3 more layers of noodles, eggplant slices, tomato sauce, and basil, omitting the basil from the last top layer.
3. Cover the baking sheet with aluminum foil; bake for 50 minutes. After 50 minutes, uncover and bake for about 10 minutes or until bubbling.
4. Let cool for about 10 minutes, slice, and then sprinkle with the remaining 1/4 cup of basil.
5. Serve with any remaining tomato sauce.

Chicken and Zucchini Fritters with Avocado Dip

Serves: 4

Prep. Time: 20 minutes

Cook Time: 30 minutes

Nutrition Facts per Serving: Calories 280; Total Fat 13.8g; Saturated Fat 3.1g;

Cholesterol 91mg; Sodium 199mg; Potassium 1377mg; Total Carbohydrates 29.9g; Dietary Fiber 6.2g; Sugars 4.6g; Protein 14.3g; Vitamin A 76%; Vitamin C 178%; Calcium 12%; and Iron 22%

Ingredients:

- 1 avocado, small-sized, mashed
- 1 tablespoon fresh basil, chopped
- 2 eggs
- 3 tablespoons flour, gluten-free
- 4 1/2 cups zucchini, grated, excess liquid squeezed out
- 4 slices toast, gluten-free
- 50 grams cooked chicken breast, finely shredded
- 8 cups salad

Directions:

1. In a large-sized bowl, combine the flour, eggs, zucchini, and chicken, and mix well.
2. In another bowl, combine the basil and avocado for the dip.
3. Grease a frying pan with oil and heat on medium-high heat. Scoop tablespoons worth of fritter mix into the frying pan; cook both sides of the fritters until they are golden. Repeat the process to make 12 fritters.
4. Serve with salad, toast, and dip.

Chicken Pot Pie
Servings: 8

Prep. Time:

Cook Time:

Nutrition Facts per Serving: Calories 231; Total Fat 7.4g; Saturated Fat 2.4g; Cholesterol 47mg; Sodium 892mg; Potassium 304mg; Total Carbohydrates 28.0g;

Dietary Fiber 5.0g; Sugars 6.7g; Protein 13.5g; Vitamin A 107%; Vitamin C 19%; Calcium 5%; and Iron 15%

Ingredients:

- 8 refrigerated biscuits
- 3 cups frozen peas – do not thaw
- 3 carrots, large-sized, peeled, diced
- 2 stalks celery, diced
- 2 cups chicken stock
- 2 cloves garlic, minced
- 190 grams chicken breast, diced into small pieces
- 1/4 cup fresh parsley, chopped finely
- 1/4 cup flour
- 1/4 cup cream OR half-and-half
- 1 teaspoon salt

- 1 teaspoon pepper
- 1 teaspoon dried thyme OR 2 teaspoons fresh thyme
- 1 tablespoon olive oil
- 1 tablespoon butter
- 1 egg, lightly beaten
- 1 cup onion, chopped

Directions:

1. Preheat the oven to400F.
2. Put the oil and the butter in a large-sized cast-iron skillet or other oven-safe skillet and heat on medium. Add the carrots, celery, onion, and thyme; cook until the vegetables start to soften.
3. Add the garlic; cook for 2 minutes more, careful not to burn the garlic. Season with pepper and salt and then blend in the flour – it will be thick. Cook for 1-2 minutes, then whisk in the cream or half-and-half; cook, constantly stirring, until the mixture is thick.
4. Add the chicken and bring the mixture to a boil. Simmer for 5 minutes.
5. Add the peas and parsley. Top the mixture with the biscuits and brush with the beaten egg.
6. Transfer the skillet into the oven and bake for about 20-25 minutes – keep an eye on to biscuit tops to prevent them from burning.

7. Remove the skillet from the oven. Let stand for a couple of minutes. Enjoy!

Zucchini Noodles, Shiitake Mushrooms, and Tomato Sauce
Serves: 2

Prep. Time: 10 minutes

Cook Time: 40 minutes

Nutrition Facts per Serving: Calories 403; Total Fat 28.7g; Saturated Fat 4.2g; Cholesterol 20mg; Sodium 462mg; Potassium 1391mg; Total Carbohydrates 29.9g; Dietary Fiber 7.9g; Sugars 15.1g; Protein 14.0g; Vitamin A 56%; Vitamin C 129%; Calcium 8%; and Iron 11%

Ingredients:

- 3 1/2 ounces shiitake mushrooms, remove stems and then slice
- 20 1/2 ounce canned peeled whole tomatoes, chopped
- 2 zucchini, medium-sized
- 1/4 teaspoon salt
- 1/2 tablespoon extra-virgin olive oil
- 1 teaspoon extra-virgin olive oil
- 1 sweet Vidalia onion, peeled and then cut into half
- 3 tablespoons extra-virgin olive oil

- 53 grams cooked chicken, shredded
- Salt and pepper, to taste

Directions:

1. In a large-sized saucepan, put the tomatoes. Add the onion, 3 tablespoons olive oil, and 1/4 teaspoon salt. Bring to a rapid boil on medium-low heat and then reduce the heat to low. Simmer for about 30-40 minutes. When the simmering is done, remove the onion from the saucepan. Using a wooden spoon or a potato masher, mash the tomatoes. Taste and if needed, season with more salt.
2. Spiralize the zucchini into noodles and put into a large-sized mixing bowl. Drizzle with 1/2 tablespoon olive oil and set aside.
3. Toss the shiitake mushrooms with pepper and salt and drizzle with 1 teaspoon extra-virgin olive oil.
4. Heat a large-sized skillet or pot on medium heat. Add the zucchini noodles; cook for about 3 to 5 minutes or until tender, stirring often.
5. When the zucchini is cooked, transfer into a colander and drain excess liquid. When drained, put the zucchini into a mixing bowl. Add 1/2 cup tomato sauce and toss to coat.
6. Divide the zoodles between 2 bowls or plates. Top with the mushrooms and the shredded chicken.

Notes: Store any unused sauce in airtight container and keep in the refrigerator for up to 1 week. Use with more zoodles.

Cauliflower Chicken Fried Rice
Serves: 2

Prep. Time: 25 minutes

Cook Time: 30 minutes

Nutrition Facts per Serving: Calories 471; Total Fat 35.2g; Saturated Fat 29.7g;

Cholesterol 15mg; Sodium 822mg; Potassium 1218mg; Total Carbohydrates 30.1g; Dietary Fiber 11.2g; Sugars 13.1g; Protein 14.4g; Vitamin A 194%; Vitamin C 236%; Calcium 11%; and Iron 14%

Ingredients:

- 500 grams cauliflower, grated into "rice"
- 5 tablespoons coconut oil
- 40 grams ground chicken
- 3 teaspoons soy sauce, gluten-free
- 2 stalks celery, chopped
- 1/4 teaspoon red pepper flakes
- 1/3 cup dried cranberries
- 1/2 cup peas
- 1 teaspoon fresh ginger, grated
- 1 teaspoon fish sauce
- 1 cup baby carrots, chopped

- 1/2 medium-sized onion, chopped
- Salt and pepper, for seasoning

Directions:

1. Put 1 tablespoons coconut oil in a medium-sized sauté pan and heat over medium-high heat.
2. Add the ground chicken and cook until no longer pink and cooked. Season with 1/2 teaspoon ginger, 1 teaspoon soy sauce, red pepper flakes, pepper, and salt.
3. Put 2 tablespoons coconut oil into a large-sized sauté pan and heat on medium-high heat. Add the peas, carrots celery, onions, 1/2 teaspoon ginger, and 1 teaspoon soy sauce. Sauté for about 3 to 5 minutes or until the veggies are softened.
4. Pour the veggie mix into sauté pan with. Add the cranberries and stir to mix.
5. Add the remaining coconut oil in the large-sized skillet. Add the cauliflower and sauté over medium-high heat for about 5 minutes or until the cauliflower gets a bit browned and season with salt and pepper.
6. Let the cauliflower rice sit in the skillet and flip using a spatula couple of times. Pour the chicken-veggie mixture and mix to combine. Pour in the remaining 1 teaspoon soy sauce and fish sauce and toss to combine. Serve.

Fennel and Roasted Eggplant Pizza
Servings: 4

Prep. Time: 30 minutes

Cook Time: 5 minutes

Nutrition Facts per Serving: Calories 399; Total Fat 26.2g; Saturated Fat 8.7g; Cholesterol 40mg; Sodium 617mg; Potassium 653mg;Total Carbohydrates 30.7g; Dietary Fiber 6.8g; Sugars 6.7g; Protein 14.4g; Vitamin A 9%; Vitamin C 20%; Calcium 32%; and Iron 13%

Ingredients:

- 1 eggplant, small-sized, sliced into 1/4-inch thick
- 1 fennel bulb, small-sized, sliced lengthwise and then halved
- 1/2 bulb garlic
- 2 pizza crusts (I used Udi's thin and crispy)
- 2 tablespoons pine nuts
- 3 1/2 tablespoons extra-virgin olive oil, divided
- 3 mint leaves
- 3/4 cup ricotta
- 4 ounces feta
- Kosher salt and black pepper, to taste

- Small handful fennel fronds

Directions:

1. Preheat the oven to 400F. Line a baking sheet with aluminum foil and then grease the foil.
2. Put the eggplant rounds and the fennel on the prepared baking sheet. Drizzle 2 tablespoons oil over the fennel and eggplant, and then season with pepper and salt. Drizzle the top of the garlic bulbs with 1/2 tablespoon oil and wrap the half bulb of garlic with aluminum foil.
3. Put the baking sheet in the oven and put the foil wrapped garlic directly on the oven rack.
4. Roast for 15 minutes or until the fennel and the eggplant are golden brown on the edges. Leave the garlic in the oven and continue roasting for about 10 minutes more or until buttery and softened.
5. Put the feta cheese, ricotta cheese, 3 cloves of roasted (removed from their paper shell), mint, and pepper to taste into a food processor; process until smooth.
6. Spread the feta cheese mixture evenly between the 2 pizza crusts. Divide and scatter the eggplant and fennel between the pizzas. Garnish with the pine nuts, remaining roasted cloves, and fennel fronds, and drizzle with 1 tablespoon olive oil.

7. Put the pizzas into baking sheet, put in the oven, and bake for about 5 to 7 minutes or until the edges are golden browned.
8. Remove from the oven. Serve.

Grilled Zucchini and Eggplant Parmesan
Serves: 4

Prep. Time: 20 minutes

Cook Time: 10 minutes

Nutrition Facts per Serving: Calories 204; Total Fat 11.4g; Saturated Fat 3.3g; Cholesterol 11mg; Sodium 989mg; Potassium 945mg; Total Carbohydrates 20.0g; Dietary Fiber 9.2g; Sugars 11.4g; Protein 10.0g; Vitamin A 11%; Vitamin C 34%; Calcium 6%; and Iron 10%

Ingredients:

- 1 3/4 cups tomato sauce, your favorite
- 1 piece (1 3/4 pounds) eggplant
- 1 zucchini, large-sized
- 1/2 teaspoon fresh ground black pepper
- 1/2 teaspoon kosher salt
- 10 large-sized basil leaves
- 2 tablespoons olive oil
- 3 ounces fresh mozzarella, thinly sliced

Directions:

1. Preheat a grill to medium heat.
2. Slice the eggplant into 1/2-inch round slices, making a total of 12 slices. In a crosswise manner, slice the zucchini into halves and then cut each half into 1/4-inch slices, making a total of 8 slices.
3. Put the zucchini and eggplant slices into a baking sheet and brush both sides of the veggies with olive oil and then season with pepper and salt.
4. Grill the veggies for about 4 minutes each side for the eggplant and 3 minutes each side for the zucchini until tender, but not overcooked.
5. During the last 30 seconds of grilling the eggplants, divide the mozzarella cheese evenly between the eggplant slices. Close the barbecue lid and cook for 30 seconds or until the mozzarella cheese is melted.
6. Lay 1 eggplant round with cheese on each 4 plates. Top each with 2 tablespoons tomato sauce. Divide ½ of the basil into 4 portions. And put a portioned basil on top of each tomato sauce and then top with each with a zucchini slice. Continue stacking in following the order, ending with an eggplant slice and tomato sauce.
7. Spoon any remaining tomato sauce around each eggplant zucchini stack. Serve immediately.

Tofu Fajitas and Guacamole Crema
Serves: 6

Prep. Time: 10 minutes

Cook Time: 35 minutes

Nutrition Facts per Serving: Calories 286; Total Fat 19.5g; Saturated Fat 3.7g; Cholesterol 2mg; Sodium 686mg; Potassium 487mg; Total Carbohydrates 22.0g; Dietary Fiber 5.8g; Sugars 4.5g; Protein 10.2g; Vitamin A 26%; Vitamin C 104%; Calcium 18%; Iron 12%

Ingredients:

For the vegetables and tofu:

- 10 ounces tofu, squeezed dry for 10 minutes between 2 plates topped with something heavy while you prepare the marinade
- 1 white onion, large-sized, sliced
- 1 red pepper, sliced
- 1 green pepper, sliced

For the marinade

- 1 cup fresh cilantro leaves
- 1 teaspoon cumin

- 1 teaspoon dried basil
- 1 teaspoon dried cilantro (or dried coriander)
- 1 teaspoon dried oregano
- 1 teaspoon fresh cracked black pepper
- 1 teaspoon red pepper flakes
- 2 limes, juice only
- 2 teaspoons sea salt
- 4 cloves garlic
- 4 tablespoons olive oil

For the guacamole crema:

- 1 avocado
- 1 cup fresh cilantro, stems and leaves
- 1 lime, juice only
- 2 cloves garlic
- 2 tablespoons red onion, chopped
- 3/4 cup Greek yogurt, plain
- Sea salt, to taste

For assembly:

- 1 cup cheddar cheese, shredded, optional
- 6 small-sized whole-wheat tortillas

Directions:

1. Preheat the oven t 425F.
2. While the tofu is being pressed, prepare the marinade. Put all of the marinade ingredients into a food processor and pulse until you have and even consistency, but not a puree.
3. Line a large-sized baking dish with aluminum foil.
4. Slice the tofu into bite-sized pieces and put into the prepared baking dish. Add the onions and peppers. Pour the marinade over the top.
5. Put the baking dish in the oven and cook for 10 minutes. Remove the baking dish, toss the tofu and the vegetables, and then return into the oven. Increase the oven temperature to 500F and cook for 25 minutes more.
6. While the tofu and veggies are cooking, prepare the guacamole crema. Put all the guacamole crema ingredients into a blender and then blend until completely smooth.
7. To assemble, divide the tofu and veggie between tortillas. Divide and drizzle the guacamole crema between the guacamole. Divide and sprinkle the cheese over each. Wrap the tortillas up.

Vegan Ratatouille

Serves: 4

Prep. Time: 15 minutes

Cook Time: 1 hour

Nutrition Facts per Serving: Calories 206; Total Fat 8.2g; Saturated Fat 1.2g; Cholesterol 16mg; Sodium 522mg; Potassium 718mg; Total Carbohydrates 24.7g; Dietary Fiber 10.0g; Sugars 14.3g; Protein 11.8g; Vitamin A 41%; Vitamin C 58%; Calcium 9%; and Iron 14%

Ingredients:

- 1 can (15 ounces or 425 grams) crushed tomatoes
- 1 eggplant
- 1 tablespoon fresh Basil, chopped
- 1 teaspoon Herbs de Provence OR mixed 1/4 teaspoon oregano, 1/4 teaspoon rosemary, and 1/2 teaspoon thyme
- 1 white onion, large-sized
- 1 zucchini
- 1/2 teaspoon crushed red pepper flakes
- 1/2 teaspoon salt
- 1/4 teaspoon black pepper
- 2 cloves garlic, minced
- 2 tablespoons olive oil, divided

- 3 Roma tomatoes
- 85 grams ground chicken, cooked

Directions:

1. Preheat the oven to 350F or 176C.
2. In a 6x9-inch baking pan, put the crushed tomatoes, basil, garlic, pepper flakes herbs, pepper, and salt and stir to combine.
3. Slice the tomatoes, eggplant, zucchini, and onion into 1/4-inch thick round slices. If some of the veggie slices are wider than the others, cut them into halves so they are the same height when they are stacked.
4. In alternate layers, layer the sliced vegetables on top of the tomato mix, placing them standing straight.
5. Brush the top of the vegetables with 1 tablespoon of olive oil.
6. Put the baking dish in the oven and bake for 1 hour or until the veggies are tender.

Coconut Curry Cauliflower

Serves: 3

Prep. Time: 20 minutes

Cook Time: 20 minutes

Nutrition Facts per Serving: Calories 580; Total Fat 50.0g; Saturated Fat 34.0g; Cholesterol 15mg; Sodium 1108mg; Potassium 1081mg; Total Carbohydrates 25.8g;

Dietary Fiber 7.9g; Sugars 11.8g; Protein 12.2g; Vitamin A 25%; Vitamin C 114%; Calcium 7%; and Iron 28%

Ingredients:

- 1 can (15-ounce) diced tomatoes
- 1 can (15-ounce) full-fat coconut milk
- 1 head cauliflower, cut into medium-sized florets
- 1 jalapeno pepper, seeds removed and minced
- 1 onion, small-sized, diced
- 1 tablespoon fresh ginger, grated
- 1/4 cup red curry paste
- 2 tablespoons vegetable oil
- Kosher salt and fresh ground black pepper

- 57 grams cooked chicken, shredded

Directions:

1. Put the oil in a Dutch oven or a large-sized pot and heat over medium heat.
2. Add the jalapeno and onion and cook for about 3 minutes or until softened.
3. Add the ginger and cook, stirring, for about 1 minute or until fragrant.
4. Add the cauliflower and pour in 1/2 cup water. Season with pepper and salt and bring to a boil. When boiling reduce the heat to a simmer and cook for about 10-15 minutes or until the cauliflower is just fork tender.
5. Divide between 3 bowls. Divide the chicken and top on each serving.

Roasted Vegetable Salad and Avocado Dressing
Serves: 4

Prep. Time: 30 minutes

Cook Time: 40 minutes

Nutrition Facts per Serving: Calories 466; Total Fat 35.9g; Saturated Fat 6.0g;

Cholesterol 9mg; Sodium 926mg; Potassium 1110mg; Total Carbohydrates 29.7g; Dietary Fiber 10.4g; Sugars 6.5g; Protein 14.0g; Vitamin A 240%; Vitamin C 260%; Calcium 10%; and Iron 17%

Ingredients:

- 4 ounces mixed greens
- 3/4 pound butternut squash
- 3/4 pound Brussels sprouts, hulled and halved
- 3 tablespoons olive oil
- 2 teaspoons dried oregano
- 1 teaspoon salt
- 1 teaspoon black pepper
- 1 red bell pepper, roughly chopped
- 120 grams canned tuna, drained, for serving

For the avocado dressing:

- 1 avocado
- 1 garlic clove, small-sized
- 1 lime, juice only
- 1/2 teaspoon salt
- 1/4 cup olive oil
- 1/4 teaspoon black pepper

Directions:

1. Preheat the oven to 400F and 200C.
2. In a large-sized bowl, mix the Brussels sprouts, butternut squash, bell pepper, salt, dried oregano, pepper, and olive oil until the vegetables are coated evenly.
3. In a single layer, transfer the veggies into a baking sheet. Put the baking sheet in the oven and roast for 40 minutes.
4. To make the dressing, put the avocado, lime juice, garlic, olive oil, pepper, and salt into a food processor or blender; process or blend until the mixture is creamy and light.
5. To serve, divide the mixed greens among 4 plates. Divide the roasted veggies between the plates. Divide and spoon the avocado dressing over each serving. Divide the tuna and sprinkle on top of each serving.